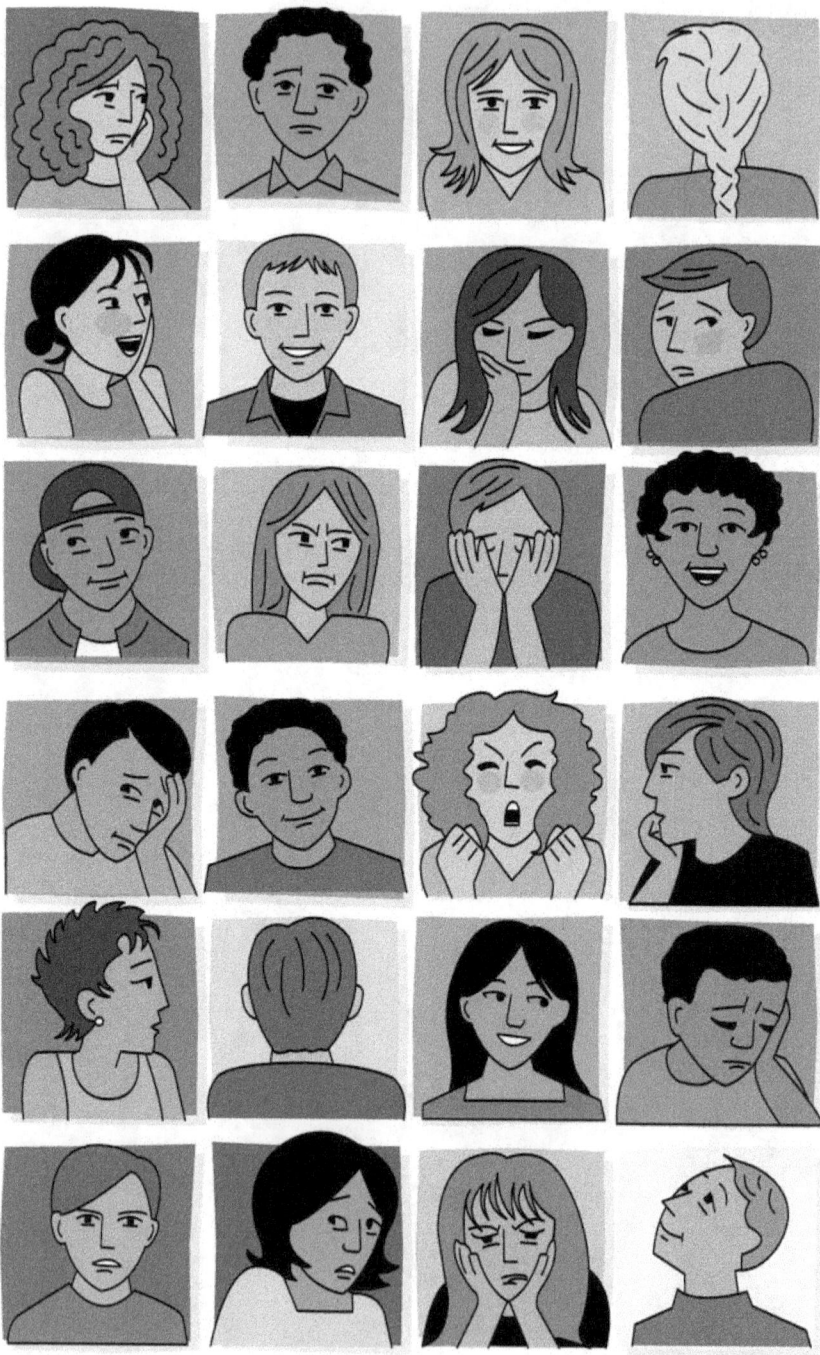

This Booklet Is For You.

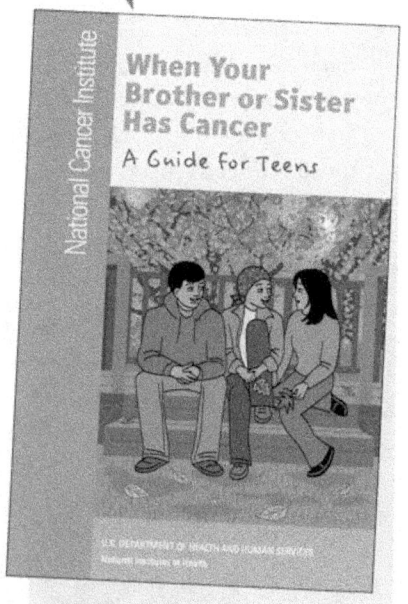

If your brother or sister has cancer, this booklet is for you.

In this booklet you will:

→ Hear from other teens who—like you—have a brother or sister with cancer

→ Find out what has helped them

→ Get ideas about people to talk with when you're upset or feel all alone

→ Learn a little about cancer and how it's treated.

This booklet can't give you all the answers, but it can help you prepare for some of the things you might face.

There is a team of people working hard to help your brother or sister get better. You should know that there are also many people available to help you. No one should go through this alone.

Free copies of this booklet are available from the National Cancer Institute (NCI). To learn more about cancer or to request this booklet, visit NCI's Web site (www.cancer.gov). You can also call NCI's Cancer Information Service at 1-800-4-CANCER (1-800-422-6237) to order the booklet or talk with an information specialist.

How To Use This Booklet

You may want to read the booklet from cover to cover. Or maybe you'll just read those sections that interest you most. Some teens pull out the booklet now and again when they need it. You may want to share this booklet with others in your family. It might help you bring up something that has been on your mind. You could ask people in your family to read a certain chapter and then talk about it together.

We've put words that may be new to you in **bold.** Turn to the glossary at the end of this booklet for their definitions.

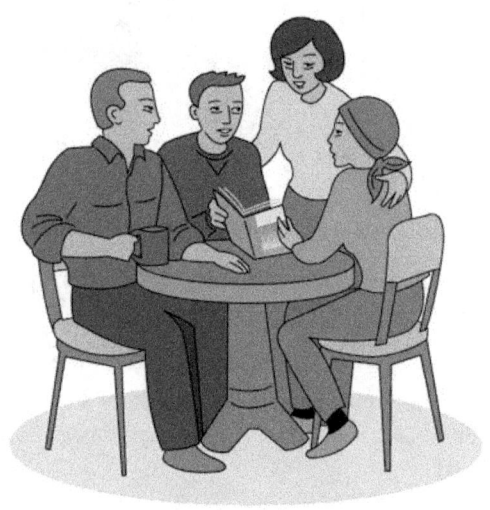

Wherever you go,

go with all your heart.

—Confucius

Table of Contents

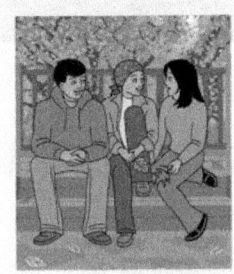

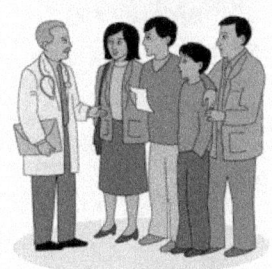

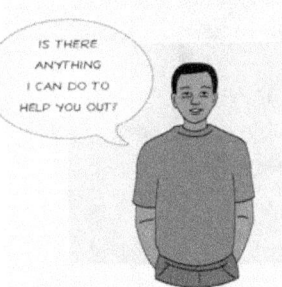

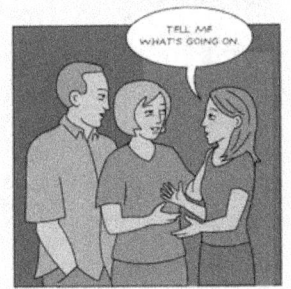

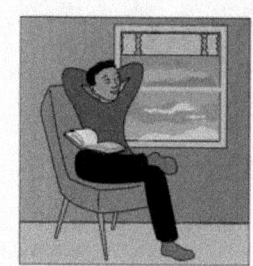

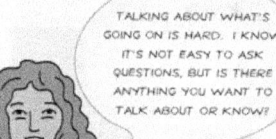

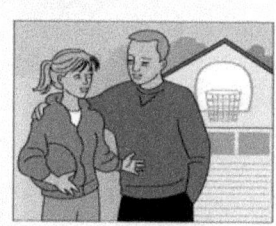

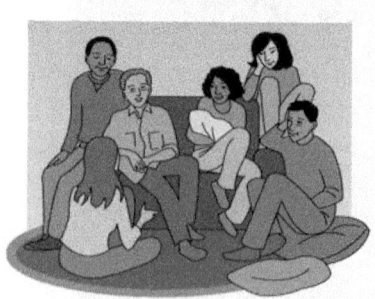

Chapter 1

You've Just Learned That Your Brother or Sister Has Cancer

You've just learned that your brother or sister has cancer. You may have a lot of emotions—feeling numb, afraid, lonely, or angry. One thing is certain—you don't feel good.

For now, try to focus on these facts:

"This is so unreal. I thought only old people got really sick—not little kids. My brother Jason has cancer, and he is only 10 years old. We found out last week, and it hasn't even sunk in yet. I wake up every morning thinking this is just a bad dream."
—Liza, age 15

→ Many kids survive cancer. You have good reason to be hopeful that your brother or sister will get better. Today, as many as 8 in 10 kids diagnosed with cancer survive their illness. Many go on to live normal lives. That's because scientists are discovering new and better ways to find and treat cancer.

→ You're not alone. Right now it might seem like no one else in the world feels the way you do. In a way you're right. No one can feel exactly like you do. But it might help to know that there are other kids who have a brother or sister with cancer. Talking to others may help you sort out your feelings. Remember, you are not alone.

→ **You're not to blame.** Cancer is a disease with many causes, many of which doctors don't fully understand. But your brother or sister did not get cancer because of anything you did, thought, or said.

→ **You can't protect, but you can give comfort.** Sometimes you'll be strong for your brother or sister, and sometimes your brother or sister will be strong for you. It's okay to talk about how hard it is and even cry together.

→ **Knowledge is power.** It can help to learn more about cancer and cancer treatments. Sometimes what you imagine is actually worse than the reality.

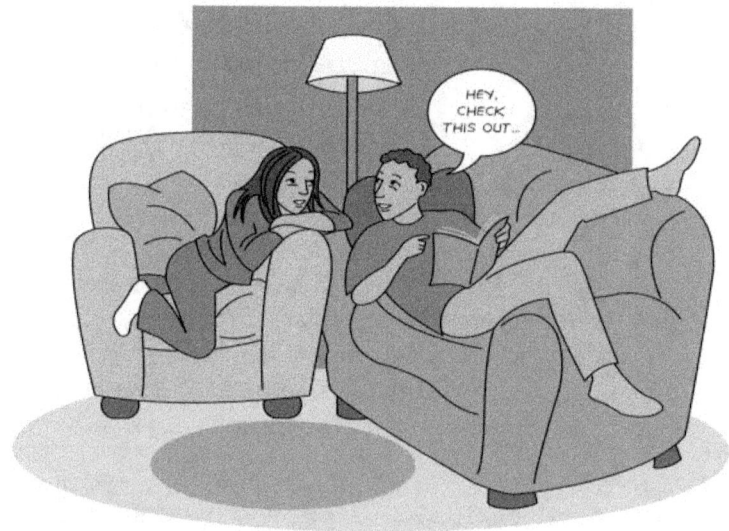

The gem cannot be polished without friction, nor man perfected without trials.

—Chinese proverb

Your Feelings

As you deal with your **sibling's** cancer, you may feel lots of different emotions. Some of the emotions you may feel are listed below.

Check off all the feelings you have today:

Scared

- [ ] My world is falling apart.
- [ ] I'm afraid that my brother or sister might die.
- [ ] I'm afraid that someone else in my family might catch cancer. (They can't.)

I feel scared because:

_____

_____

It's normal to feel scared. Some of your fears may be real. Others may be based on things that won't happen. And some fears may lessen over time.

Guilty

- [ ] I feel guilty because I'm healthy and my brother or sister is sick.
- [ ] I feel guilty when I laugh and have fun.

I feel guilty because:

_____

_____

You might feel guilty about having fun when your sibling is sick. This shows how much you care about them. But you should know that it is both okay and important for you to do things that make you happy.

7

Angry

☐ I am mad that my brother or sister is sick.

☐ I am angry at God for letting this happen.

☐ I am angry at myself for feeling the way I do.

☐ I am mad because I have to do all the chores now.

I am angry because:

_____

_____

Anger often covers up other feelings that are harder to show. If having cancer in your family means that you can't do what you like to do and go where you used to go, it can be hard. Even if you understand why it's happening, you don't have to like it. But, don't let anger build up inside. Try to let it out. And when you get mad, remember that it doesn't mean you're a bad person or you don't love your sibling. It just means you're mad.

"Sometimes, I feel mad at my brother for having cancer. I know that's not right, and he can't help it. But it has changed everything. My mom and dad don't talk about anything but him, and neither does anyone else. It's just not fair."

—Tyree, age 13

"At night both my parents go in my sister's room to talk and be with her. I'm the youngest, and I need them, too. Do they both have to be with her every night?"

—Sarah, age 14

Neglected

☐ I feel left out.

☐ I don't get any attention any more.

☐ No one ever tells me what's going on.

☐ My family never talks anymore.

I feel neglected because:

_____

_____

When your brother or sister has cancer, it's common for the family's focus to change. Your parents don't mean for you to feel left out. It just happens because so much is going on. You may want to tell your parents how you feel and what you think might help. Try to remember that you are important and loved and that you deserve to feel that way, even though you might not get as much attention from your parents right now.

Lonely

- ☐ My friends don't come over anymore.
- ☐ My friends don't seem to know what to say to me anymore.
- ☐ I miss being with my brother or sister the way we used to be.

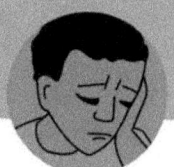

I feel lonely because:

_____

_____

We look at some things that may help you deal with changes in friendships in Chapter 9, and at things others have done to stay close to their siblings in Chapter 7. For now, try to remember that these feelings won't last forever.

Embarrassed

- ☐ I'm sometimes embarrassed to be out in public with my sibling because of how they look.
- ☐ I feel silly when I don't know how to answer people's questions.

I feel embarrassed because:

_____

_____

It can help to know that other teens also feel embarrassed. So do their siblings. In time it gets easier, and you will find yourself feeling more comfortable.

I'm feeling upset that my brother or sister is getting all the attention.

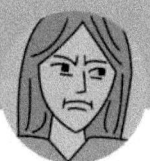

Jealous

I feel jealous because:

_____

_____

Even if you understand why you are getting less attention, it's still not easy. Others who have a brother or sister with cancer have felt the same way. Try to share your feelings with your parents and talk about what you think might help.

What You're Feeling Is Normal

There is no one "right" way to feel. And you're not alone—many other teens in your situation have felt the same way. Some have said that having a brother or sister with cancer changes the way they look at things in life. Some even said that it made them stronger.

"I feel so bad for my big sister. She's sick all the time. She used to be the one I looked up to, and now everything has changed. Now, she looks to me for support. I feel like I'm having to grow up so fast."

—Riley, age 12

11

Dealing With Your Feelings

A lot of people are uncomfortable sharing their feelings. They
ignore them and hope they'll go away. Others choose to act
cheerful when they're really not. They think that by acting upbeat
they won't feel sad or angry anymore. This may help for awhile,
but not over the long run. Actually, holding your feelings inside
can keep you from getting the help that you need.

Try these tips:

→ **Talk** with family and friends that you feel close to. You owe it
to yourself.

→ **Write** your thoughts down in a journal.

→ **Join a support group** to meet other kids who are facing
some of the same things you are. Or meet with a counselor.
We'll learn more about these options in Chapter 10.

It is probably hard to imagine right now, but, if you let yourself,
you can grow stronger as a person through this experience.

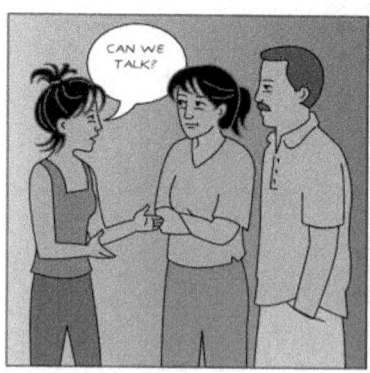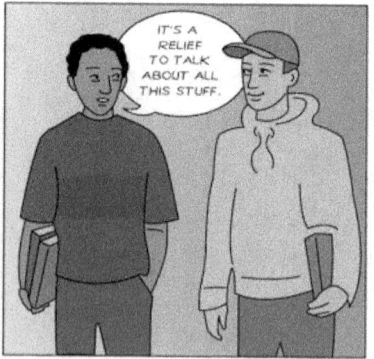

"When my dad comes home from being with my sister at the hospital all day, he is so grumpy. One day I just asked him why he always seemed so mad at me. He got quiet and said he's so worried and stressed that even little things set him off . . . and that being on edge isn't fair to me and my other sister. Hearing what was going on inside my dad's head made me realize how tough this whole situation is for him, too. It made me feel a lot closer to him, instead of so alone and mad." —Kevin, age 15

"It's a pain to do the dishes by myself all the time. Before he got sick it was my brother's job to wash and my job to dry. We had a system." —Justin, age 17

"I had to give up going to drill team after school because I had to be home to take care of my little sisters while Mom took Jay to the doctors." —Becky, age 16

13

"I was so scared when I found out that my brother had cancer. In the movies cancer always seems so terrible. Then I realized that I didn't really know that much about cancer. I started reading and learned a lot. I found out that most kids survive cancer."

—Rashid, age 14

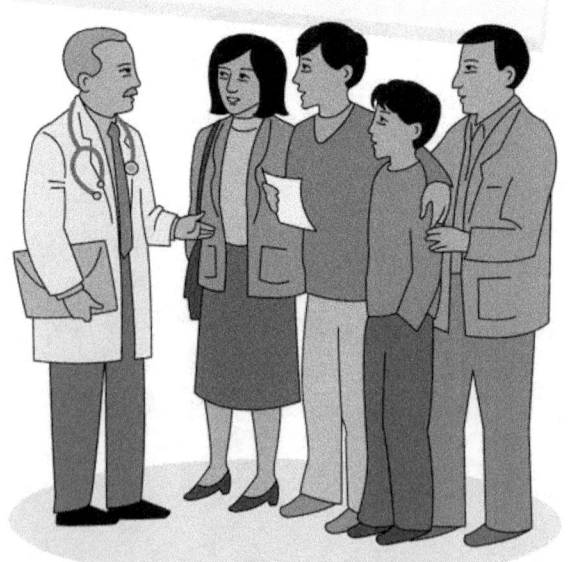

Chapter 2

Learning About Cancer

Learning about cancer and your brother's or sister's treatment can help you feel less afraid. Some of what you have seen or heard about cancer may not apply. Most people feel better when they know what to expect.

Here are a few facts to remember:

→ Nothing you did, thought, or said caused your brother or sister to get cancer.

FACTS

→ You can't catch cancer from another person.

→ Scientists are finding many new and better ways to find and treat cancer.

→ Most kids survive cancer.

"I got really mad at Chrissy one day. She wouldn't let me ride her bike. I got mad and said, 'I wish you were dead.' Now she has leukemia. I thought maybe it was my fault. I was scared to tell anyone because then they'd all know what I did and be mad. But my dad heard me crying one night, and got me to talk to him. He said it wasn't my fault or anybody's that Chrissy has cancer."
—Katie, age 13

What Is Cancer?

Doctors have found more than 100 different types of cancer. Cancer is a group of many related diseases that begin in **cells**, the body's basic unit of life. To understand cancer, it's helpful to know what happens when normal cells become cancer cells.

Normally, cells grow and divide to make more cells only when the body needs them. This orderly process helps to keep the body healthy. Sometimes, however, cells keep dividing when new cells aren't needed. These extra cells form a mass of **tissue**, called a growth or **tumor.** Tumors can be **benign** or **malignant:**

→ **Benign tumors aren't cancerous.** They can often be removed and don't spread to other parts of the body.

→ **Malignant tumors are cancerous.** Cells in these tumors are abnormal and divide and grow without control or order. They can invade and damage nearby tissues and spread to organs in other parts of the body. The spread of cancer from one part of the body to another is called **metastasis.**

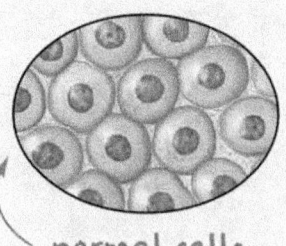

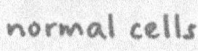

normal cells

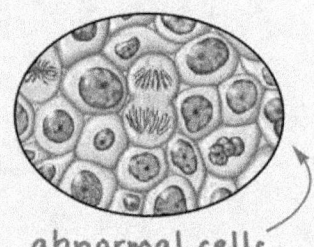

abnormal cells

Most cancers are named for the organ or type of cell in which they begin. For example, cancer that begins in the bone is called bone cancer. Some cancers do not form a tumor. For example, **leukemia,** which is the most common cancer among children, is a cancer of the **bone marrow** and blood.

Why Do Children Get Cancer?

The causes of most cancers aren't known. Cancer among children does not happen that often. Scientists are still trying to learn more about why some kids get cancer and others don't.

Will I Get Cancer, Too?

If you are worried that you may get cancer, you should know that most cancers don't run in families. You and your parents can talk to a doctor for more information.

Can Doctors Cure Cancer?

Every year scientists discover better ways to treat cancer. That means many people are successfully treated for cancer. However, doctors are careful not to use the word "cure" until a patient remains free of cancer for several years. Cancer treatment may cause a **remission,** which means that the doctor can't find signs of cancer. But sometimes the cancer comes back. This is called a **relapse** or **recurrence.** Whether your brother or sister will be cured of cancer depends on many things. No booklet can tell you exactly what to expect. It is better to talk with your parents and your sibling's doctor or nurse.

Where to go for more information

To learn more about the type of cancer your brother or sister has, visit the National Cancer Institute's (NCI) Web site (http://www.cancer.gov). You can also call NCI's Cancer Information Service at 1-800-4-CANCER (1-800-422-6237) to talk with an information specialist. All calls are free and confidential.

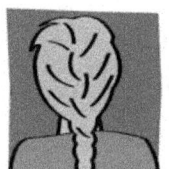 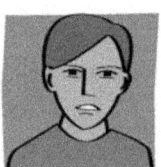 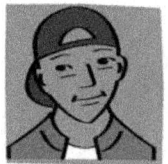 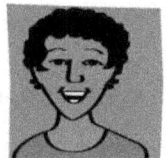

He who is not everyday

conquering some fear

has not learned

the secret of life.

—Ralph Waldo Emerson

Chapter 3

Cancer Treatment

You may want to know what to expect during your brother's or sister's cancer treatment.
This chapter briefly explains different treatments. It talks about how they work and their **side effects.** You will probably have more questions after reading this chapter.
It may help to talk with your parents. Or ask if you can talk with your sibling's nurse or social worker.

"Rachel had all this beautiful hair. But during treatment, she'd wake up and find hair all over her pillow. It would also fall out when she combed or washed it. I could hear her crying in the bathroom. One day Mom helped her shave her head. Then we bought and decorated some bandanas together. They look good on her. My sister is my hero."
—Lauren, age 12

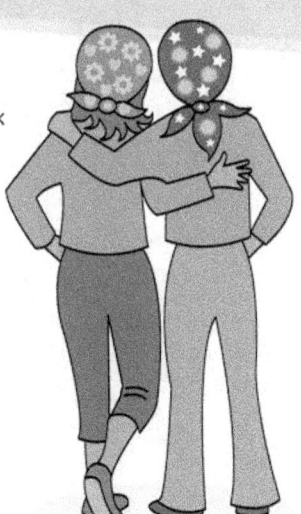

How Does Treatment Work?

Cancer treatment aims to get rid of cancer cells. The type of treatment your brother or sister will be given depends on:

→ The type of cancer

→ Whether the cancer has spread

→ Your sibling's age and general health

→ Your sibling's medical history

→ Whether the cancer is newly diagnosed or has recurred.

Remember that there are more than 100 different types of cancer, and each type is treated differently.

Treatment follows a **protocol,** which is a treatment plan. But even if two people have the same type of cancer and the same treatment plan, it may not work the same way for both of them. This is because people's bodies can react differently to treatment. Most children with cancer are treated at large pediatric cancer centers in **clinical trials.** A clinical trial is a study that helps show how, for example, a promising anticancer drug, a new test, or a possible way to prevent cancer affects the people who receive it.

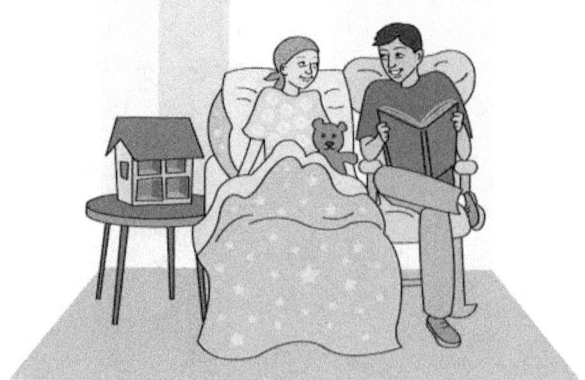

What Are Treatment Side Effects?

Side effects happen because the cancer treatment targets fast-growing cells. Cancer cells are fast growing, but so are normal cells like the ones in the digestive tract and hair, for example. The treatment can't tell the difference between fast-growing normal cells and fast-growing cancer cells. That's why people sometimes get sick to their stomach and lose their hair when they have **chemotherapy** (one type of cancer treatment).

Some side effects, like feeling sick to the stomach, go away shortly after treatment, while others, like feeling tired, may last a while after treatment has ended.

Write down what treatment your brother or sister will get:

_____

_____

_____

_____

_____

Use the chart on the next two pages to find out more about different types of cancer treatment.

The chart describes six types of cancer treatment, how they're done, and some of the side effects. Your brother or sister may get one or more of these treatments. Depending on the exact treatment, they may visit the doctor during the day, or they may stay overnight in the hospital.

TREATMENT CHART			
Treatment	What is it?	How is it done?	What may happen as a result? (side effects)
Surgery Also called an operation	The removal of all or part of a solid tumor	A surgeon operates to remove the cancer. Drugs are used so that the patient is asleep during surgery.	• Pain after the surgery • Feeling tired • Other side effects, depending on the area of the body and the extent of the operation.
Radiation therapy Also called radiotherapy	The use of high-energy rays or high-energy particles to kill cancer cells and shrink tumors	Radiation may come from a machine outside the body or from radioactive material placed in the body near the cancer cells.	• Feeling tired • Red or blistered skin • Other side effects, depending on the area of the body and the dose of radiation.
Chemotherapy Also called chemo	The use of medicine to destroy cancer cells	The medicine can be given as pills, through an injection (shot), or through an **intravenous (IV)** line. It is often given in cycles that alternate between treatment and rest periods.	• Feeling sick to the stomach or throwing up • Loose bowel movements or not being able to go to the bathroom • Hair loss • Feeling very tired • Mouth sores • A feeling of numbness, tingling, or burning in the hands and feet.

TREATMENT CHART *(continued)*

Treatment	What is it?	How is it done?	What may happen as a result? (side effects)
Stem cell transplantation Can be a bone marrow transplantation (BMT) or a peripheral blood stem cell transplantation (PBSCT)	The use of **stem cells** found in either the bone marrow or the blood. This repairs stem cells that were destroyed by high doses of chemo and/or radiation therapy.	Stem cell transplantation uses stem cells from the patient or from **donors**. In many cases, the donors are family members. The patient gets these stem cells through an IV line.	• The side effects can be much like those from chemo and radiation. In some cases, the side effects may be worse.
Hormone therapy	A treatment that adds, blocks, or removes **hormones** from the body. Hormone therapy is especially useful to slow or stop the growth of some types of cancers.	Hormone therapy can be given as a pill, through an injection, or through a patch worn on the skin. Sometimes surgery is needed to remove the glands that make specific hormones.	• Feeling hot • Feeling tired • Weight changes • Mood changes.
Biological therapy Also called immunotherapy	Biological therapy uses the body's own defense system (the **immune system**) to fight cancer cells.	Patients may be given medicine in pills, through an injection, or through an IV line.	• Chills/fever • Muscle aches • Weakness • Feeling sick to the stomach or throwing up • Loose bowel movements.

Your brother or sister will get tests to monitor the cancer and how the treatment is working. See Chart A in the back of this booklet for a list of some common monitoring tests.

Things To Look For

Some treatments may make your brother or sister more likely to get an infection. This happens because cancer treatment can affect the white blood cells, which are the cells that fight infection. An infection can make your brother or sister sicker. So your sibling may need to stay away from crowded places or people who have an illness that he or she could catch (such as a cold, the flu, or chicken pox).

Because of this, you may need to:

→ Wash your hands with soap and water often to keep from spreading germs

→ Tell a parent when you've been around someone who's sick or has a cold

→ Stay away from your brother or sister if you get sick.

The Waiting

It's hard to wait to see how well the treatment will work. Your brother's or sister's doctor may try one treatment, then another. One day your brother or sister may feel a lot better, and the next day or week they may feel sick again. Treatment can go on for months or sometimes years. This emotional roller coaster is hard on everyone.

During this time, remember that the treatment is working to stop the cancer and make your brother or sister better. For more information about the people who will be treating your brother or sister, see Chart B in the back of this booklet.

Want To Visit?

Close to home

If your brother or sister is in a hospital near you, you may be able to visit. Learn ahead of time how your sibling is doing and what to expect. You can read together, draw, play games, or sit and talk. Some teens also want to help care for their brother or sister. Ask the nurse what you can do if you are interested.

"I looked forward to the times I got to visit my big sister when she was in the hospital. Sometimes it was really sad to see Tara in bed because she looked so weak. But I am glad I went. Now my sister is home, so I get to see her again." —Allie, age 14

Far from home

When your brother or sister is getting treatment far from home, you may not be able to visit them as often. It will help you both to stay in touch. Talk on the phone. You can also send cards, letters, or pictures back and forth.

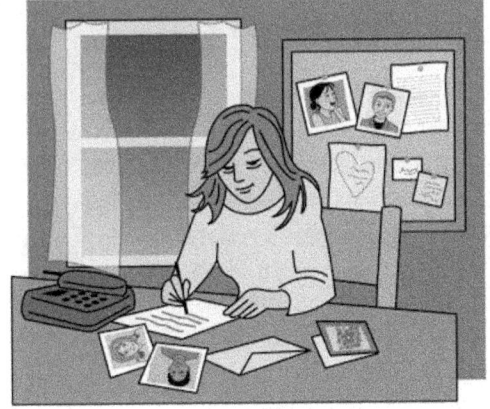

Your Own Ups and Downs During Treatment

During your brother's or sister's treatment, you may go through a whole new range of feelings.

Does this sound like how you feel sometimes?

→ I feel frustrated.

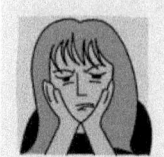

→ I feel left out.

→ I feel invisible—my sibling is getting all the attention.

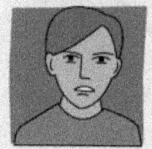

→ I feel like treatment has gone on so long.

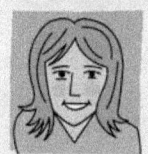

→ I am so sad that my sibling is so sick.

→ I wonder why this is happening to our family.

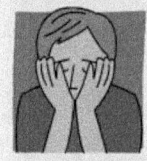

→ Some days I want to know all the details about treatment. Other days I just want to forget it ever happened.

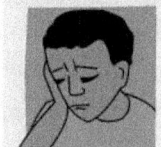

All of these feelings are natural. Try to share your thoughts with your friends, parents, or another trusted adult. This time can be tough on every member of your family. Talking things through can help when you are feeling left out, sad, or confused.

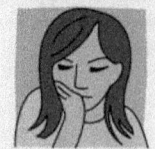

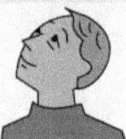

Where to go for more information

To learn more about cancer treatments, visit the NCI Web site (http://www.cancer.gov). Look for the booklets *Chemotherapy and You,* and *Radiation and You,* among others. You can also call the NCI's Cancer Information Service at 1-800-4-CANCER (1-800-422-6237) to talk with an information specialist. All calls are free and confidential.

"One day I went to the clinic with my brother for his treatment. I saw the machine that he gets radiation from. I got to meet his doctor and nurses and see lots of other kids with cancer. I still wish Jake's treatment was over, but I feel better knowing more about what is going on." —Matthew, age 15

Where Do Kids Get Treated for Cancer?

Most kids get treated at cancer treatment centers that are just for children and teens. There may be a center near you. Or your brother or sister may have to get treatment in another city or state. Your parent and your sibling, or your whole family, may go live in a new city during treatment.

Who Can Answer My Other Questions?

Ask your parents or another trusted adult any questions that you have. Ask if you can go along and maybe talk with a doctor or nurse when your parents take your brother or sister to the doctor.

To make things easier:

➔ Make a list of questions and bring the list with you.

➔ Ask people to explain things using simple words.

"At first I didn't ask any questions, although I had a lot of them. I thought people would think I was really dumb, but now I know it really helps to ask." —Brad, age 15

➔ Ask for the information to be repeated.

➔ Ask the doctor or nurse to show you things on a model or draw a picture.

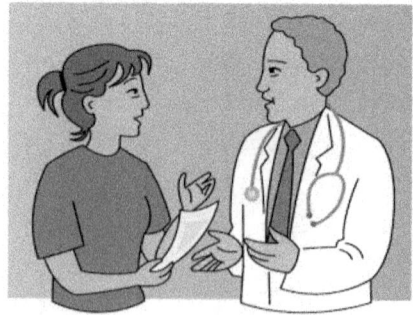

Questions you might want to ask

→ What kind of cancer does my brother or sister have?

→ Will my brother or sister get better?

→ What are the chances I will get this kind of cancer, too?

Questions about the treatment

→ What kinds of treatment will my brother or sister get? Will there be more than one?

→ How do people feel when they get this treatment? Does it hurt?

→ How often is this treatment given? How long will it last?

→ Does the treatment change how people look, feel, or act?

→ What happens if the treatment doesn't work?

→ Where are treatments given? Can I come along?

Write down your own questions:

_____

_____

_____

_____

_____

_____

It's okay to ask these questions more than once.

"I was surprised to find out about stem cell donation because I didn't think I would have any role in my sister's treatment. So when I was asked to be a donor, I felt like it was a chance to help her in an important way. At first I had a lot of questions. A nurse was the person that helped me the most."
—Ethan, age 17

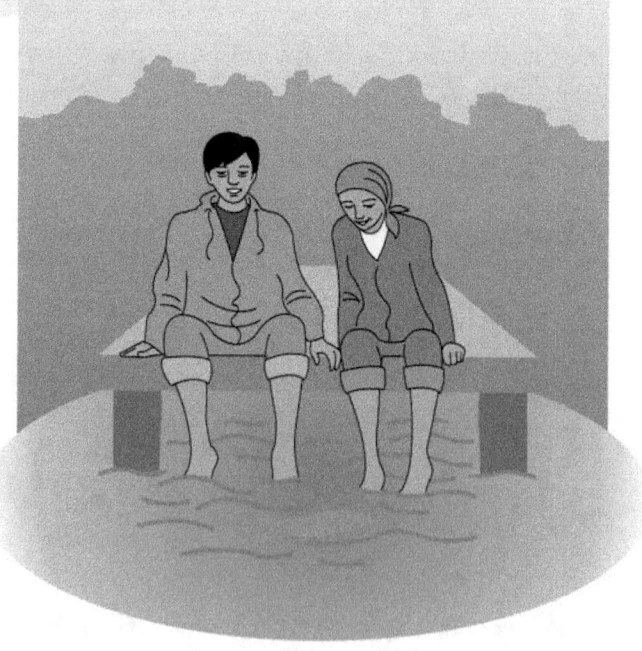

Do what you can, with what you have,

Chapter 4

Becoming a Stem Cell Donor

In Chapter 3 we listed bone marrow transplantation (BMT) and peripheral blood stem cell transplantation (PBSCT) as possible cancer treatments. Only some children with cancer get these treatments. If your sibling is going to receive one of them, you may find it helpful to read this chapter. Otherwise, you can skip it.

Why Do Some Cancers Need Bone Marrow or Stem Cell Transplants?

Sometimes very high doses of chemo and/or radiation therapy are used to treat cancer. These treatments destroy cancer cells but also wipe out good cells, like stem cells.

FACT

What Are Stem Cells?

Stem cells make the blood cells needed to carry oxygen to all the parts of the body (red blood cells), fight infection (white blood cells), and prevent bleeding (platelets). Most are found in the bone marrow—the spongy material that fills the inside of bones. Some are also found in the bloodstream.

How Transplants Work

Healthy stem cells collected from a brother or sister are **transplanted** into the sibling with cancer. The stem cells travel to the bone marrow and make new red blood cells, white blood cells, and platelets. These new cells help your brother or sister recover from the cancer treatments.

Who Can Be a Donor?

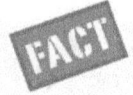

A stem cell donor can be a brother or sister or a volunteer (from the National Marrow Donor Program®). Stem cells can also be collected from the patient's own body prior to cancer treatment and stored for later use.

Facts about donors:

→ A donor is a person whose stem cells match those of the person with cancer. Not everyone is a match.

→ A patient's brother or sister is more likely to match than someone who is not related.

→ In one out of four cases, a brother or a sister is a good match.

→ When no one in the family is a match, the medical team can look for a volunteer donor from around the world.

Thoughts From Teens Who Were Donors

→ "I was scared. No doubt about it—the thought of being a donor made me nervous 'til I knew what was going to happen."

→ "I didn't feel like I had a choice until my parents said it was up to me to decide if I wanted to do this or not."

→ "I felt my big brother and my whole family were counting on me for this to work. I am glad that it did!"

Courage is the first of human qualities because it is

What If I'm Asked To Be a Donor?

If you agree to be a donor, the doctor will do a special blood test to find out whether you are a match for your brother or sister. The test will show whether your stem cells are a good match or not.

What If I'm Not a Match?

You may be tested and find out that you are not a match. You may feel disappointed or that you are letting your brother or sister down. It's important to know that it's not your fault if you are not a match. While it's natural for your family to feel down, no one should be upset with you.

"I was so disappointed that neither my sister Heather or I were a match for our little sister Taylor who has cancer. No one blamed us—but it was still hard. Now the doctors are trying to find a match from other donors." —Caitlin, age 13

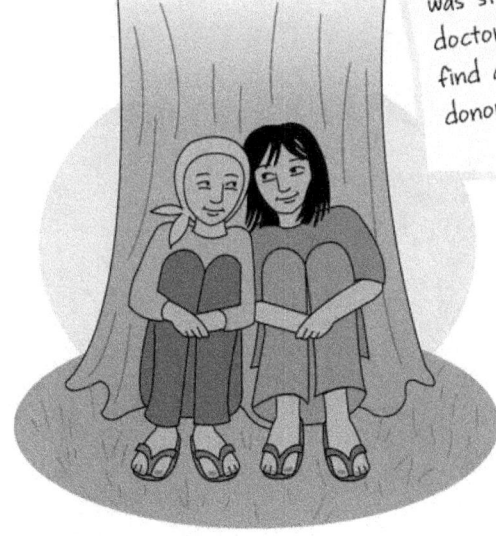

Don't be afraid to ask questions about anything that you don't understand or feel comfortable about. Write down some of your questions:

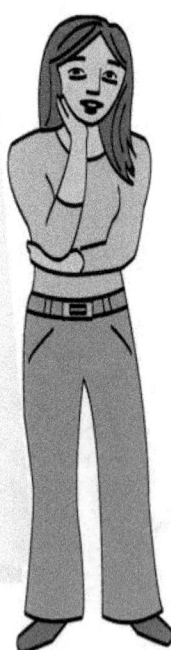

"The doctor told me I was a match for my brother Chris. My mom said it was my choice—I did not have to be a donor if I didn't want to. But even though I was kind of nervous, I wanted to do it. Chris's doctor met with us to explain what would happen. I hope this will help my brother." —Amber, age 15

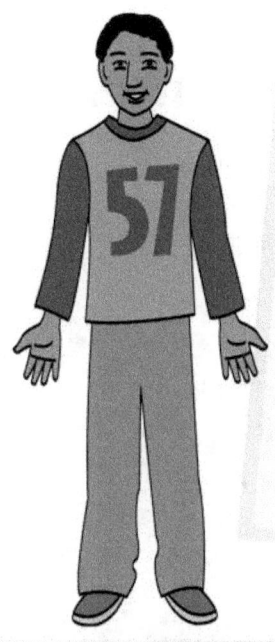

"It didn't hurt as much as I thought it would to be Jada's donor. Before I knew it, I was playing softball again. My advice to other kids who want to be donors is to ask questions—lots of them. It would have helped me to be more prepared. I really didn't know what to expect."

—Anthony, age 16

What happens during the transplant?

For a bone marrow transplantation (BMT), the doctors collect stem cells from your bone marrow. Before the doctor collects the stem cells, you will get medicine to help you fall asleep. Then the doctor will put a needle into your hip bone to collect the bone marrow. You won't feel pain from the needle because you will be asleep. Afterwards, you may be a little stiff or sore for a couple of days at the place where the needle went in.

For a peripheral blood stem cell transplantation (PBSCT), the doctors collect stem cells from your blood. A doctor will take blood from you, usually through a vein in your arm. Your blood will go through a machine that removes the stem cells. Then your blood is put back into you. The stem cells are stored and later given to your sibling through a **transfusion.**

What If the Transplant Doesn't Work?

No one can guarantee that the transplant will make your sibling get better, but the chance to help your brother or sister can be very rewarding. It can help you feel more involved. However, it can be difficult if the transplant doesn't work. Know that it wasn't your fault. You did what you could, and no one should blame you.

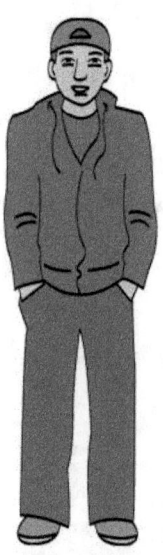

"I turned out to be a match for my brother David. The bad news was that the transplant didn't help my brother. I felt like I had really let him down. But David told me not to feel bad about it. He told me how much it meant to him that I even gave it a try."

—Jason, age 15

What about other questions that I have?

Ask any questions that you have. Doctors, nurses, and social workers can all help you. So can your parents. Your family can also get more information from the National Marrow Donor Program®. It is an organization that keeps a list of volunteer donors and transplant centers. Call 1-800-MARROW-2 (1-800-627-7692) or go to http://www.marrow.org.

Chapter 5

What Your Brother or Sister May Be Feeling

Just like everyone else, your brother or sister may be worried, scared, or confused. They may also feel tired and sick because of the treatment. Some kids feel embarrassed because treatment has changed the way they look and feel. You both may be having a lot of the same feelings.

Look at the World Through Your Brother's or Sister's Eyes

Knowing how your brother or sister might be feeling could help you figure out how to help, or at least understand where they are coming from.

Here are a few things young people with cancer have felt:

Afraid

Depending on how old your brother or sister is and how they react to tough situations, they may be more or less afraid.

"It's scary to learn that you have cancer. Will the treatment hurt? Who are all these doctors and nurses prodding at me and asking me questions? I don't like not knowing what will happen. I don't like not knowing if I will get better." —Tamara, age 13

Sad or Depressed

People with cancer sometimes can't do things they used to do. They may miss these activities and their friends. Feeling sad or down can range from a mild case of the blues to **depression,** which a doctor can treat.

"I hate it that I can't do a lot of the things I used to do. I miss hanging out with my friends. I never thought I would say this, but I even miss school. A lot of the time I just don't want to talk at all, and when I do, I can't be cheerful and happy all the time."
—Ryan, age 15

"I admit it. I am not nice a lot of days. I feel ticked off. People get on my nerves. I'm like—why is this happening to me? Some days I just feel mad about everything."
—Jeremy, age 16

Angry

Cancer and treatment side effects can cause your brother or sister to be mad or grumpy. Anger sometimes comes from feelings that are hard to show, like being afraid, being very sad, or feeling helpless. Chances are your sibling is angry at the disease, not at you.

"Everything is different now that I have cancer. It's like the whole family just stopped doing what they were doing. I know my sisters can't be happy about that. They have to do all the chores. My older sister had to stop cheerleading so she could take care of my little sister after school. I feel guilty that I brought this on." —Nicole, age 14

Guilty

Your brother or sister may feel guilty that they caused changes in your family's life. But just as you did not cause this situation to happen, neither did your brother or sister.

Hopeful

There are many reasons for your brother or sister to feel hopeful. Most kids survive cancer, and treatments are getting better all the time. Hope can be an important part of your brother's or sister's recovery.

"I keep the faith. I put up a huge sign in the living room that says 'If you have to be blue, be a bright blue!' My three brothers and I used all these blue colored markers and we decorated it with glitter. I have to keep believing that I will get cured. It is what keeps me going."
—Julie, age 16

All of these feelings are normal for a person living with cancer. You might want to share this list with your sibling. Ask them how they are feeling.

Dear Diary,

What is going on? Everything is changing so fast. Six months ago I was the little sister ready to start high school. Now I am the most adult one in the family. Since Jill got sick, Mom is a mess—sad and stressed all the time. She thinks we don't see, but we do. All our time is spent going to Jill's doctor visits. Dad works day and night and all Jill does is lie around and listen to music. I know the cancer makes her mad, but does she have to shut me out? Is my family ever going to get back to normal again?

—Beth, entry from September 18th

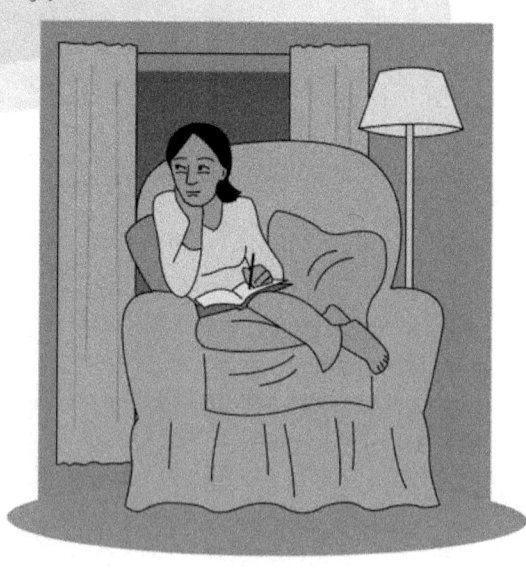

Work is love made visible. —Kahlil Gibran

Chapter 6

Changes in Your Family

Changing Routines and Responsibilities

Your family may be going through a lot of changes. You may be the oldest, youngest, or middle child in your family. You may live with one parent or two. Whatever your family situation, chances are that things have changed since your brother or sister got sick. This chapter looks at some of these changes and ways that others have dealt with them.

Does this sound like your home?

☐ Are you doing more chores?

☐ Are you spending more time with relatives or friends?

☐ Are you home alone more?

☐ Are you asked to help make dinner or do the laundry?

☐ Are you looking after younger brothers or sisters more?

☐ Do you want to just hang out with your friends when you are needed at home?

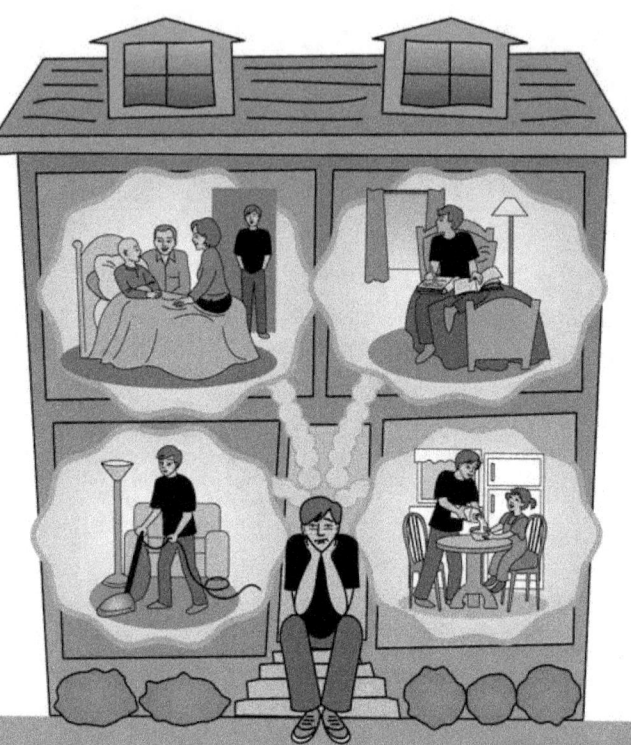

Does this sound like you?

→ Do you feel like you have to be perfect and good all the time?

→ Do you try to protect your parents from anything that might worry them?

→ Do you feel like yelling, but hold it in because you don't want to cause trouble?

No one can be perfect all the time. You need time to feel sad or angry, as well as time to be happy. Try to let your parents and others you trust know how you're feeling—even if you have to start the conversation.

Your Relationship With Your Parents

Your parents may ask you to take on more responsibility than others your age. Your parents may be spending more time with your brother or sister. You might resent it at first. Then again, you may grow and learn a lot from the experience. See Chapter 10 for tips on talking with your parents.

Touching Base When Things Are Changing

Families say that it helps to make time to talk together—even if it's only for a short time each week. Talking can help your family stay connected. Here are some things to consider when talking with:

Other brothers and sisters

→ If you are the oldest child, your younger brothers or sisters may look to you for support. Help them as much as you can. It's okay to let them know that you are having a tough time, too.

→ If you are looking to your older brother or sister for help, tell them how you are feeling. They can help, but they may not have all the answers.

Try saying something like this:

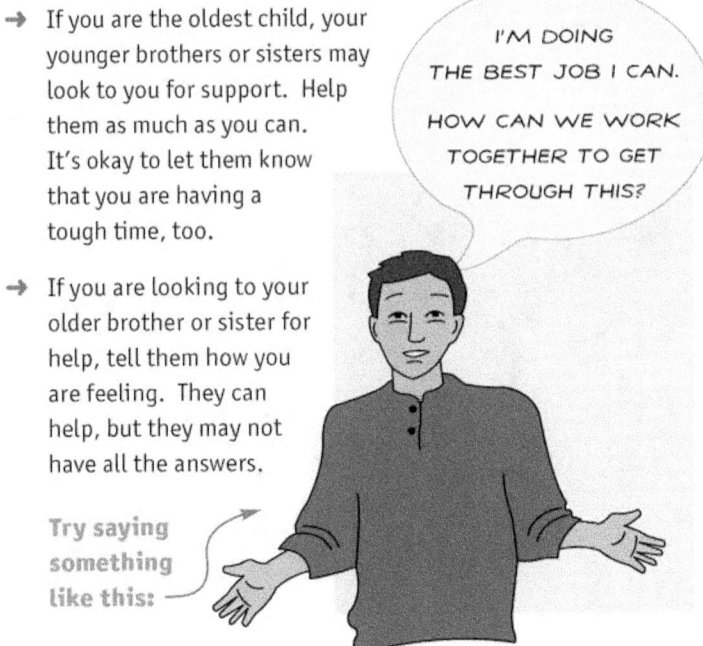

I'M DOING THE BEST JOB I CAN.

HOW CAN WE WORK TOGETHER TO GET THROUGH THIS?

Your parents

→ Expect your parents to feel some stress, just like you may. Your parents may not always do or say the right thing.

→ Try to make the most of the time you do have with your parents. Let them know how much it means to you. Maybe you can go out to dinner together, or they can come to your sports game, from time to time.

→ Sometimes you may have to take the first step to start a conversation. You may feel guilty for wanting to have your needs met—but you shouldn't. You are important and loved, too.

→ Keep talking with your parents, even though it may be hard.

Try saying something like this:

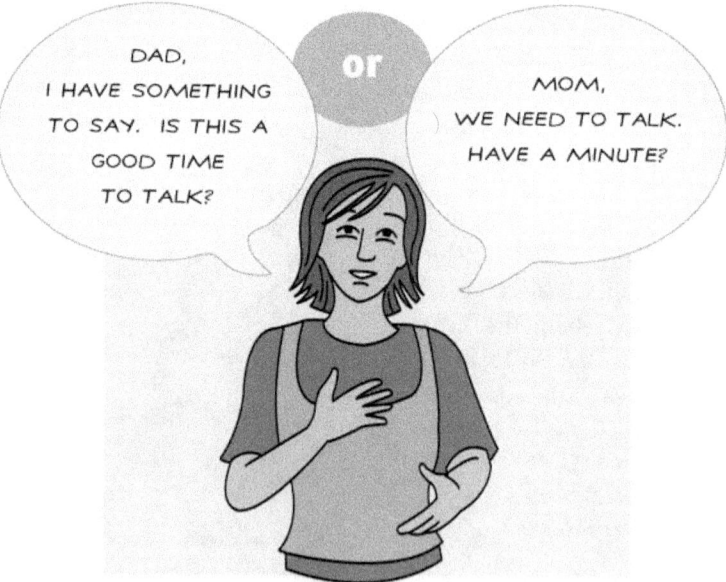

DAD, I HAVE SOMETHING TO SAY. IS THIS A GOOD TIME TO TALK?

or

MOM, WE NEED TO TALK. HAVE A MINUTE?

the dance changes. —Nigerian proverb

You may want to try saying something like this:

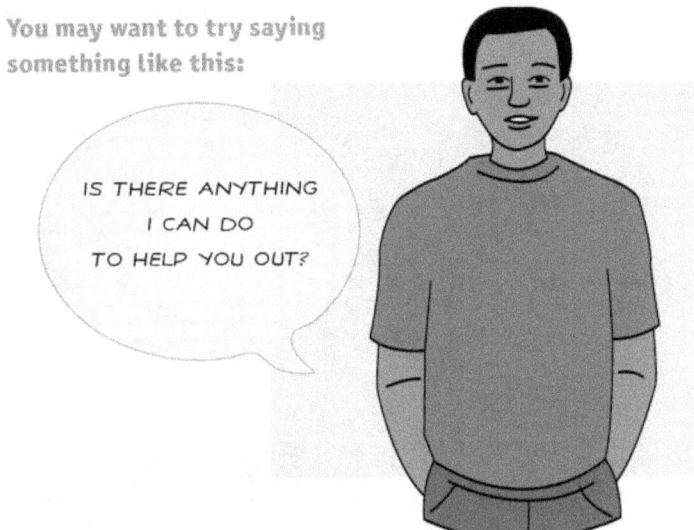

Your brother or sister with cancer

→ Your brother or sister may be sick from the treatment and want to be alone. Or maybe they feel okay and want your company.

Try saying something like this:

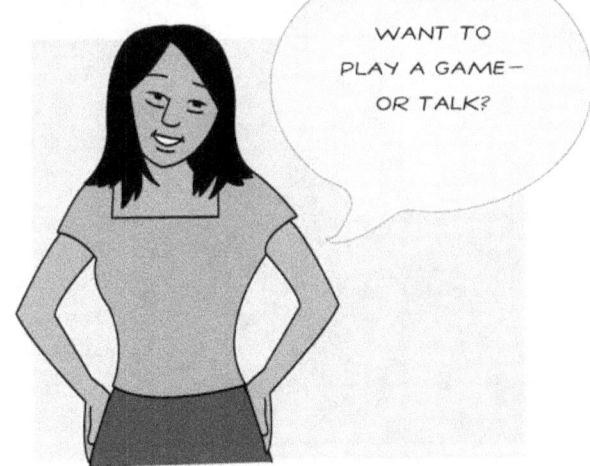

45

"I just wasn't ready for all these changes. My sister Kelly and I had always shared a bedroom. But when she got sick, she got the bedroom because Mom and Dad had to keep coming in during the night. Some nights I had to sleep on the couch in the living room. My brother Tim and I can't even have friends over as much anymore because they could bring germs when Kelly is sick. It's very different now." —Jessica, age 13

Keeping the Conversation Going

If you're used to talking openly at home, you might find that your parents aren't sharing as much anymore.

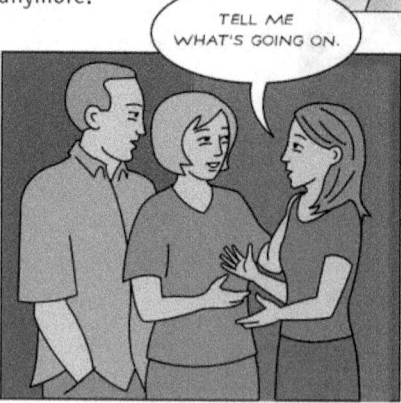

TELL ME WHAT'S GOING ON.

Maybe they're trying to protect you from bad news or unsure about what to tell you. Some teens want to know a lot, while others only want to know a little. Tell your parents how much you want to know.

Over the next few weeks or months, you may overhear parts of your parents' conversations. If what you hear confuses or scares you, talk with your parents about what you heard.

Keeping Family and Friends in the Loop

Challenge	Solution
It's getting to be too much to answer the phone all the time and tell people how your brother or sister is doing.	Ask others to help you share news of how your brother or sister is doing. Maybe a relative or family friend can be the contact person and help let others know how your brother or sister is doing. Some families use a Web site or e-mail listserv to share this information.

Getting Help When You Need It

Challenge	Solution
Your family can't keep up with the house, meals, and other activities.	Friends and neighbors often want to help make meals, clean, drive, or look after you and your siblings. Make a list with your parents of what needs to get done. Keep the list by the phone. When people ask what they can do to help, pull out the list.

Growing Stronger as a Family

Some families can grow apart for a while when a child has cancer. But there are ways to help your family grow stronger and closer. Teens who saw their families grow closer say that it happened because people in their family:

"My family wasn't really close before my sister Gina got cancer. We used to go our own way and never did much together. When Gina got sick, we started pulling together more. We talked to our pastor about how much more each day meant. Now it seems like even simple things are special—like eating dinner together as a family." —Jared, age 13

→ **Tried** to put themselves in the other person's shoes and thought about how they would feel if they were the other person

→ **Understood** that even though people reacted differently to situations, they were all hurting. Some cried a lot. Others showed little emotion. Some used humor to get by.

→ **Learned** to respect and talk about differences. The more they asked about how others were feeling, the more they could help each other.

"We all acted differently when my middle brother Terrell got cancer. My younger brother started acting like a baby again and my older brother never seems to be home. I'm the only girl and feel like I have to hold it all together for my whole family." —Keisha, age 14

48

Asking Others for Help

You and your family may need support from others. It can be hard to ask. Yet most of the time people really want to help, so don't hesitate to ask.

"Brian and I are not just brothers, we're best friends. When he got sick, it was so hard for me that I didn't feel like doing anything or talking to anyone. I felt down a lot, but I didn't let anyone know. Being at home wasn't much fun because Brian was always so sick. My math teacher noticed that I was different and asked me what was up. It's been good to have someone I can go to when I need to get things off my chest."

—Mike, age 18

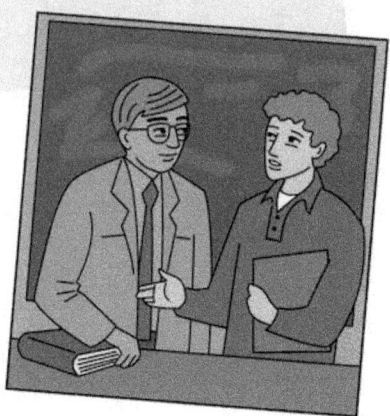

People that you or your parents may ask for help:

→ Grandparents, aunts, and uncles

→ Family friends

→ Neighbors

→ Teachers and coaches

→ People from your religious community

→ Your friends and their parents

→ School nurses and guidance counselors.

Ways people can help you:

→ Help with homework.

→ Talk with you and listen to you.

→ Give rides to school or practice.

→ Invite you over or on weekend outings.

Other things people can do to help around the house:

→ Buy groceries or run errands.

→ Make meals.

→ Mow the lawn.

→ Do chores around the house.

What are some other ways that people can help you?
List some ideas here:

_____

_____

Chapter 7

How You Can Help Your Brother or Sister

This chapter has some things that others have done to help their brother or sister. Pick one or two things you may want to try this week. Then pick a couple more next week.

"People used to call Jessie and me 'the twins.' We are 13 months apart, but we look so much alike and we were always together. Now that Jess has cancer she's lost all her hair and —well, unfortunately, people can tell us apart. Last week I decided to do something pretty drastic to show my sister how much I love her. I shaved my head! Now, I am not saying that is the right thing for all sisters to do—but it felt like the right thing for us." —Renee, age 15

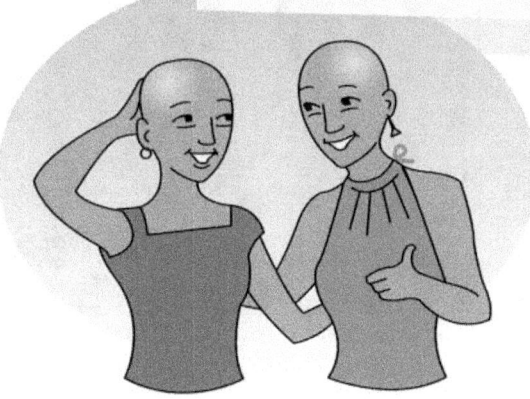

Help by Just Being There

→ **Hang out together.** Watch a movie together. Read or watch TV together. Decorate your brother's or sister's bedroom with pictures or drawings. Go to the activity room at the hospital and play a game or do a project together.

→ **Comfort one another.** Just being in the same room as your brother or sister can be a big comfort. Do what feels best for the two of you. Give hugs or say "I love you." Laugh or cry together. Talk to one another. Or just hang out in silence.

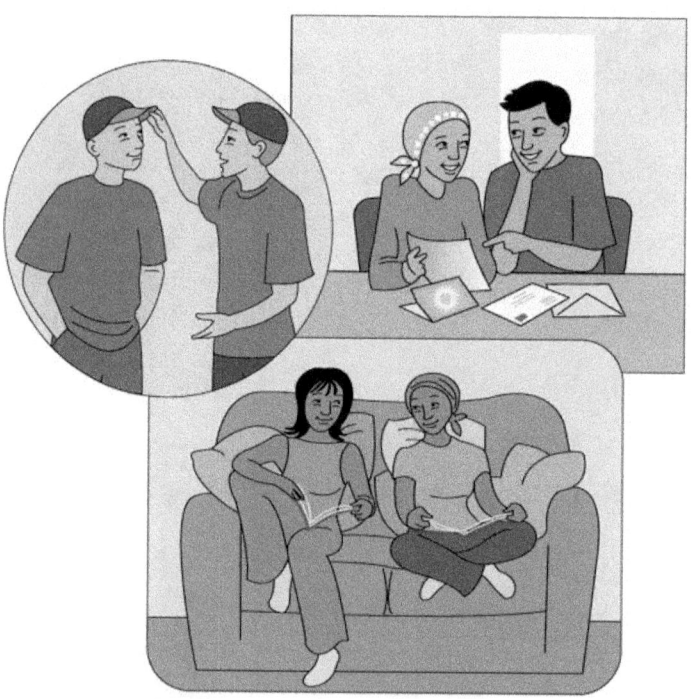

Help by Being Thoughtful

→ **Help your brother or sister stay in touch with friends.**
Ask your sibling's friends to write notes, send pictures, or
record messages. Help your brother or sister send messages
to their friends. If your brother or sister is up for it, invite
friends to hang out with them.

→ **Share a laugh.** You've probably heard that laughter is good
medicine. Watch a comedy or tell jokes together, if that is
your thing.

→ **Be patient.** Be patient with each other. Your brother or
sister may be cranky or even mean. As bad as you feel, your
brother or sister is probably feeling even worse. If you find
you are losing your cool, go for a run, read, or listen to music.

→ **Make a snack.** Make a snack for the two of you to share.
Make a picnic by putting a blanket on the porch or in the
bedroom.

→ **Buy a new scarf or hat.** Your brother or sister might like a
new hat or scarf if they have lost their hair during treatment.
Get a matching hat or scarf for yourself, too.

→ **Try to be upbeat, but be "real," too.** Being positive can
be good for you and your whole family. But don't feel like
you have to act cheerful all the time if that's not how you
really feel. Try to be yourself.

> I am only one, but I am one.
>
> I cannot do everything,
>
> but I can do something.
>
> —Edward Everett Hale

53

Help by Staying Involved

→ **Keep a journal together.** Write thoughts or poems, doodle, or put photos in a notebook. Take turns with your sibling writing in a journal. This can help you both share your thoughts when it might be hard to talk about them.

→ **Go for a walk together.** If your brother or sister feels up to it, take a walk together. Or, open a window or sit on the front porch together.

The ideas above are for those times when you have extra energy to give. Don't forget to take care of yourself, too. You deserve it. Read more about taking care of yourself in the next chapter.

Can you think of some other ways to help your brother or sister?
Make your own list here:

Chapter 8

Taking Care of Yourself

"When we found out my sister Kiana had cancer, we all seemed to focus on her—and nothing else. I was so worried that I stopped hanging out with friends and quit training for track meets. One day my mom said that giving up all these things wasn't good for me. She said it was okay to have fun and practically pushed me out the door to start going to track again. I didn't think anyone noticed me, but I'm glad my mom did! She even came to my next track meet!"
—Patrick, age 16

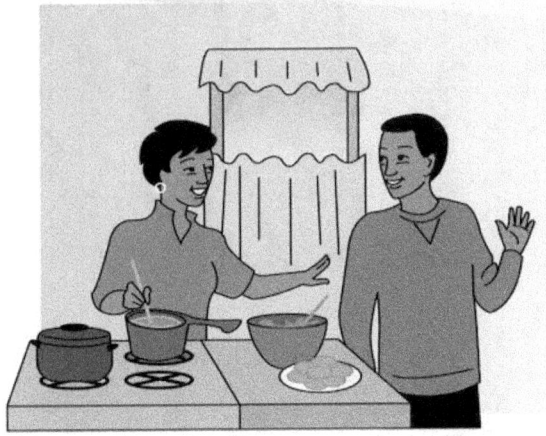

It's Important To "Stay Fit"— Both Inside and Out

You may be so focused on your sick brother or sister that you don't think about your own needs, or if you do, they don't seem important. But they are! Read this chapter to learn ways to stay balanced at a time when everything may feel up in the air.

Dealing With Stress

Stress can make you forgetful, frustrated, and more likely to catch a cold or the flu. Any way you look at it, too much stress isn't good.

Here are some tips that have worked to help other teens manage stress. In the lists on the next few pages, check one or two things to do each week.

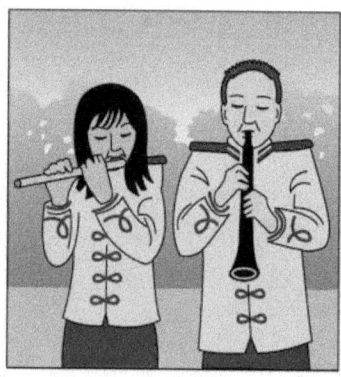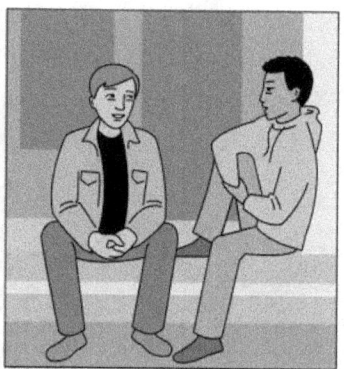

Turn your face to the sun
and the shadows fall behind you.

—Maori proverb

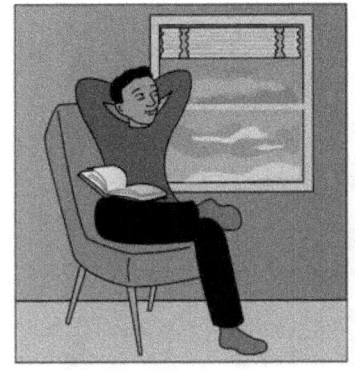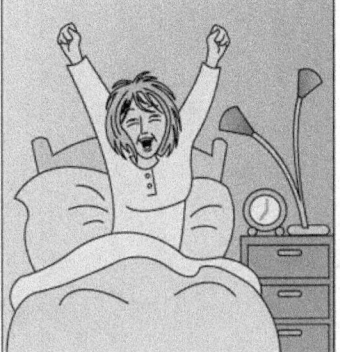

Take Care of Your Mind and Body

→ Stay connected.

- [ ] Spend some time at a friend's house.

- [ ] Stay involved with sports or clubs.

- [ ] Add your own here:

_____

→ Relax and get enough sleep.

- [ ] Take breaks. You'll have more energy and be in a better frame of mind.

- [ ] Get at least 8 hours of sleep each night.

- [ ] Pray or meditate.

- [ ] Make or listen to music.

- [ ] Add your own here:

_____

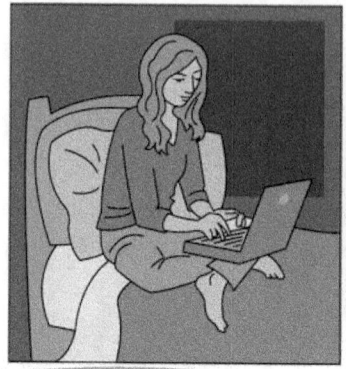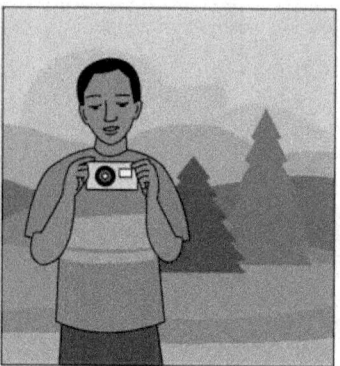

→ **Help others.**

- ☐ Join a walk against cancer.

- ☐ Plan a bake sale or other charity event to collect money to fight cancer.

- ☐ Add your own here:

  _____

→ **Avoid risky behaviors.**

- ☐ Stay away from smoking, drinking, and other risky behaviors.

→ **Put your creative side to work.**

- ☐ Keep a journal to write down your thoughts and experiences.

- ☐ Draw, paint, or take photographs.

- ☐ Read books or articles about people who have made it through difficult experiences in life. Learn what helped them.

- ☐ Add your own here:

  _____

→ Eat and drink well.

☐ Switch to caffeine-free drinks in the evening that won't keep you awake.

☐ Grab fresh fruit, whole-grain breads, and lean meats like chicken or turkey when you have a choice.

☐ Avoid foods that have a lot of sugar.

☐ Drink 6–8 glasses of water a day to help prevent fatigue.

☐ Add your own here:

_____

→ Be active.

☐ Play a sport or go for a run.

☐ Take the dog for a walk.

☐ Learn about different stretching and breathing exercises.

☐ Add your own here:

_____

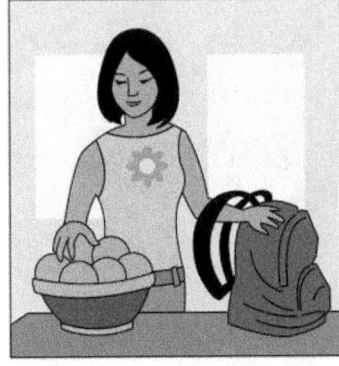
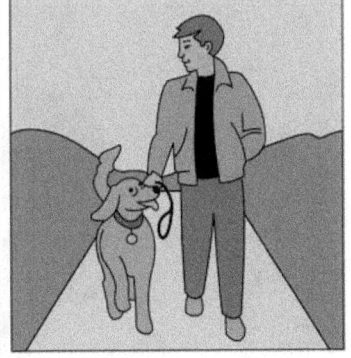

Take Steps To Keep Things Simple

Staying organized can also keep your stress level under control.
Here are some tips to get you started.

→ At home

- ☐ Make a list of things you want to do. Put the most important ones at the top.
- ☐ Make a big calendar to help your family stay on top of things.

→ At school

- ☐ Let your teachers know what's happening at home, without using it as an excuse.
- ☐ Talk to your teachers or a counselor if you are falling behind. They can help you.

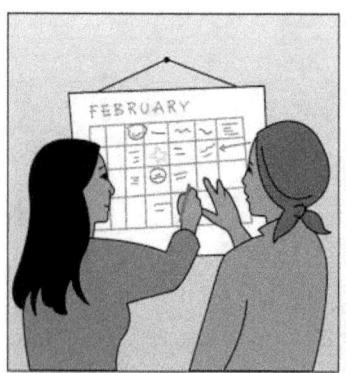 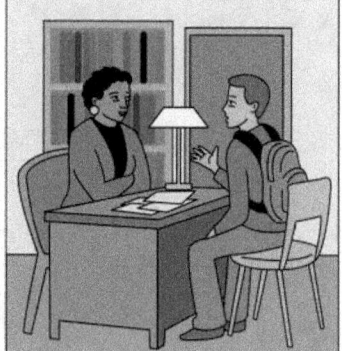

"It sounds weird—since my family didn't used to be that organized—but keeping track of everything on a calendar really helped us stay on track. It made everything feel more under control—especially when things got a little crazy." —Eric, age 17

What Else Can You Do?

The ideas listed above may help. You may also have others that would work even better. Write down your ideas below:

Get Help When You Feel Down and Out

Many teens feel low or down when their brother or sister is sick. It's normal to feel sad or "blue" during difficult times. However, if these feelings last for 2 weeks or more and start to interfere with things you used to enjoy, you may be depressed. The good news is that there is hope and there is help. Often, talking with a counselor can help. Below are some signs that you may need to see a counselor.

Are you:

- Feeling helpless and hopeless? Thinking that life has no meaning?
- Losing interest in being with family or friends?
- Finding that everything or everyone seems to get on your nerves?
- Feeling really angry a lot of the time?
- Thinking of hurting yourself?

Do you find that you are:

- Losing interest in the activities you used to enjoy?
- Eating too little or a lot more than usual?
- Crying easily or many times each day?
- Using drugs or alcohol to help you forget?
- Sleeping more than you used to? Less than you used to?
- Feeling tired a lot?

If You Answered "Yes"
To Any of These Questions...

It's important to talk to someone you trust. Going to see a counselor doesn't mean that you are crazy. In fact, it means that you have the strength and courage to recognize that you are going through a difficult time and need help. Read more about what teens who've talked with a counselor or met with a support group have to say in Chapter 10.

"It got to the point where I was feeling down all the time, like I just didn't have any energy and nothing seemed fun anymore. I even stopped hanging out with my friends. I felt like I couldn't tell anyone what was going on, not even my family. But then I started talking with a counselor and now things are getting back on track." —Jake, age 17

"My grades were slipping. I wasn't that great a student before my sister got cancer. Once she got really sick I stopped caring about school. My art teacher noticed that my drawings were different. She talked with me and helped me get an appointment with the guidance counselor. I feel like a weight's been lifted off my shoulders. I still worry about my sister, but am doing better in school now." —Ray, age 16

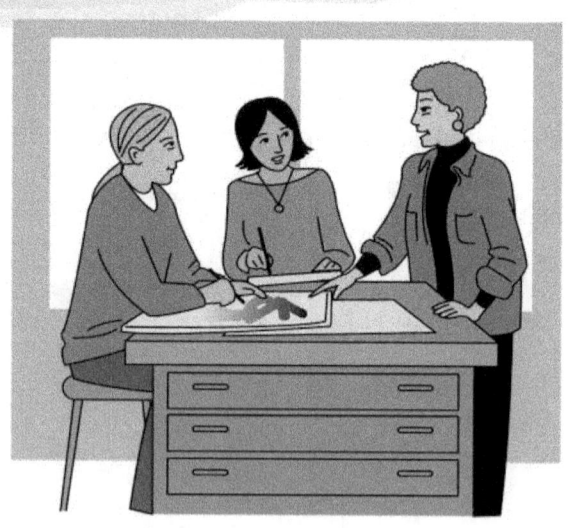

Chapter 9

You and Your Friends

Your friends are important to you, and you're important to them. In the past, you could tell them everything. Now that your brother or sister has cancer, it may seem like lots is changing—even your friendships. Here are some things to think about:

Some friends may not know what to say.

→ It's hard for some people to know what to say. They may be afraid of upsetting you. Try to be gentle with friends who don't ask how you're doing or who don't talk about your brother's or sister's cancer.

→ You may need to take the first step.

→ Try saying something like this: ⟶

"Before my big brother Trevor got cancer, my three best friends were my life. I didn't go anywhere without them. I was never really home. Things are different now. I still see my friends, but I want to hang out with Trevor a lot more now. I definitely don't take him for granted anymore. My friends keep on going like nothing has changed. And for them—nothing has." —Taylor, age 16

TALKING ABOUT WHAT'S GOING ON IS HARD. I KNOW IT'S NOT EASY TO ASK QUESTIONS, BUT IS THERE ANYTHING YOU WANT TO TALK ABOUT OR KNOW?

Some friends may ask tough questions.

→ It may be hard to answer questions about what you and your family are going through. You may want to try to help your friends understand what's going on. Or sometimes you may not feel like talking at all.

→ Try saying something like this:

→ If you don't feel like talking, try saying something like this:

"Sometimes it's hard talking about everything that's going on. If this was happening to one of my friends, I probably wouldn't know what to say to them, either. It just makes me appreciate even more the friends who have called or stopped by to hang out."
—Justin, age 16

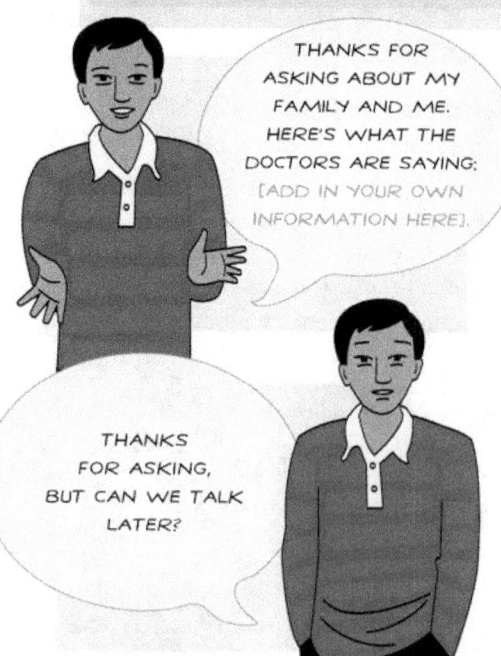

THANKS FOR ASKING ABOUT MY FAMILY AND ME. HERE'S WHAT THE DOCTORS ARE SAYING: [ADD IN YOUR OWN INFORMATION HERE].

THANKS FOR ASKING, BUT CAN WE TALK LATER?

"People asked me questions all the time. They'd say things like, 'I heard Molly isn't coming back to school this year' or 'I heard your mom was having a breakdown.' When I told them the truth, they didn't believe me. And they'd ask dumb questions like, 'Can Molly walk? Can she write?' They didn't know what was going on, and I didn't know how to answer them. I got sick of it." —John, age 14

Your friends have their own lives.

→ It may feel like your friends don't care anymore. It might seem as though their lives are moving on and yours is not. It can be hard to watch them get together with others or do things without you. They aren't facing the situation you are right now, so it may be hard for them to relate.

→ You might want to try saying something like this:

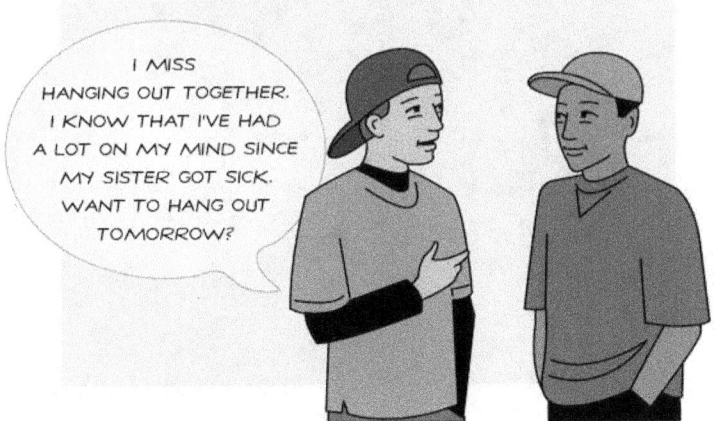

I MISS HANGING OUT TOGETHER. I KNOW THAT I'VE HAD A LOT ON MY MIND SINCE MY SISTER GOT SICK. WANT TO HANG OUT TOMORROW?

"I get the feeling my friends want me to just 'get over it' and go back to how life was before we found out my sister has cancer. But I wish they understood that sometimes I just don't feel like doing what they're doing or talking about what they're talking about. I really want to spend time with my sister."
—Max, age 15

"Now that my brother lost his hair and is so skinny, I don't want my friends to come over anymore. I don't want them to see how Tim looks. Besides, it's not easy to laugh and play at home when he's so sick." —Caroline, age 14

"My friends have been great. They love Emma like she was their own sister. It helps to know that they care."
—Angie, age 13

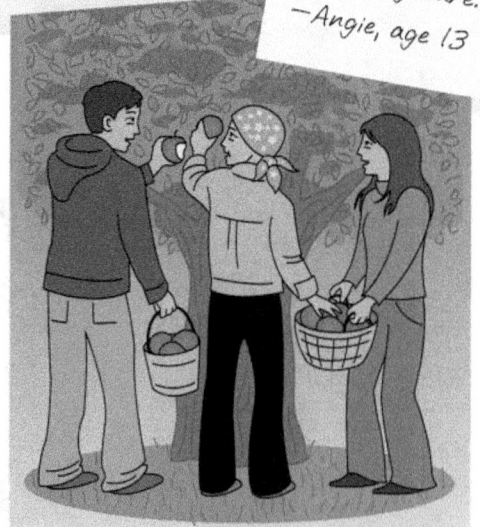

Dealing With Embarrassment

It may be hard to talk with your friends. You may feel embarrassed that your brother or sister has cancer, or that now your family is different. You may not want to tell anyone about it. But when someone in your family is sick, you really need friends you can talk with.

Having Fun and Making New Friends

Old friends:

Even though you may have a lot on your mind, you can still get together with your friends and have a good time. If you can't leave home as much, ask if your friends can come over. Make time to relax. It's both good and important for you.

Make a list of fun things you and your friends like to do together. Then do them!

New friends:

A lot is happening to you right now. Sometimes old friends move on. You may not have as much in common as you used to. The good news is that you may make new friends through this experience. Kids who used to just pass you in the halls may now ask you how you are doing. Kids who you used to be friends with may become close friends again. Be open to new friendships.

Going to **support groups** at the hospital or at school is a good way to meet new friends. Support groups can help connect you with other kids who can relate to you—because they're going through some of the same things that you are.

Dealing With Hurtful Remarks

Unfortunately, some kids may say mean things. Others speak before they think and before they get the facts. No matter the reason, it can hurt when kids make jokes or say hurtful things about you, cancer, or your brother or sister.

What can you do?

→ Ignore the comment.

→ Say, "Hey, my brother/sister has cancer. It's not funny. How would you feel if it were your brother/sister?"

→ Being bullied? Go to your teacher, principal, or guidance counselor right away.

Chapter 10

Finding Support

Don't let being afraid of the way you feel keep you from talking to your parents, a counselor, or kids in a support group.

For many people, starting to talk is difficult. Some teens don't have good relationships with their parents. Others are too embarrassed to talk about personal things. It can also just be hard to make the time to talk, with all that is going on. But you and your parents really can help each other.

"Before I went to a support group I felt like my sister's cancer was just something that I had to deal with on my own. I thought it would be dumb and depressing to talk with others who were going through the same thing as me—but it's helped a lot! I would tell other kids to find a support group for sure. Check out more than one if you don't like the first one you go to."
—Devon, age 15

TiP Don't be shy about asking for help.

You may think: "I can solve all my own problems." However, when faced with tough situations, both teens and adults need support from others!

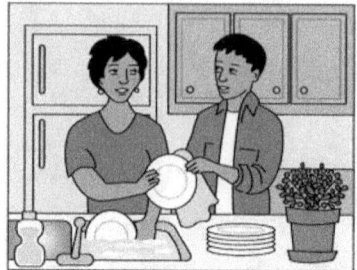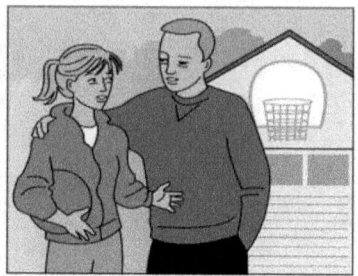

Here Are Some Tips
for Talking With Your Parents

Prepare before you talk.

STEP 1
Think about what you want to say and about some solutions to the problem.

STEP 2
Think about how your parents might react. How will you respond to them?

Find a good time and place.

STEP 1
Find a private place, whether it's your room or the front steps. Or maybe you can talk while taking a walk or shooting hoops.

STEP 2
Ask your parents if they have a few minutes to talk.

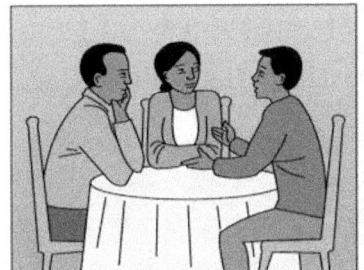
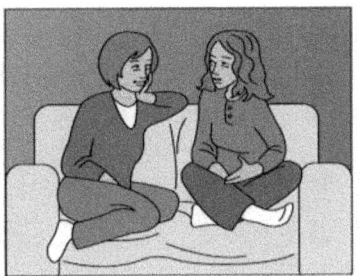

Take things slowly.

STEP 1 · · · · · · · · · · · · · · · ▶ **STEP 2**

Don't expect to solve
everything right away.
Difficult problems
often don't have
simple solutions.

Work together
to find a way through
these challenges.
Some conversations
will go better
than others.

Keep it up.

STEP 1 · · · · · · · · · · · · · · · ▶ **STEP 2**

Don't think you have to
have just one big
conversation.
Have lots of
small ones.

Make time
to talk a little each day
if you can, even if it's
just for a
few minutes.

Talking With a Counselor

Sometimes talking to friends and your parents is not enough. When you are having a hard time, it can be helpful to talk to a counselor. Friends Brice and Nick talk about what is happening in Brice's home:

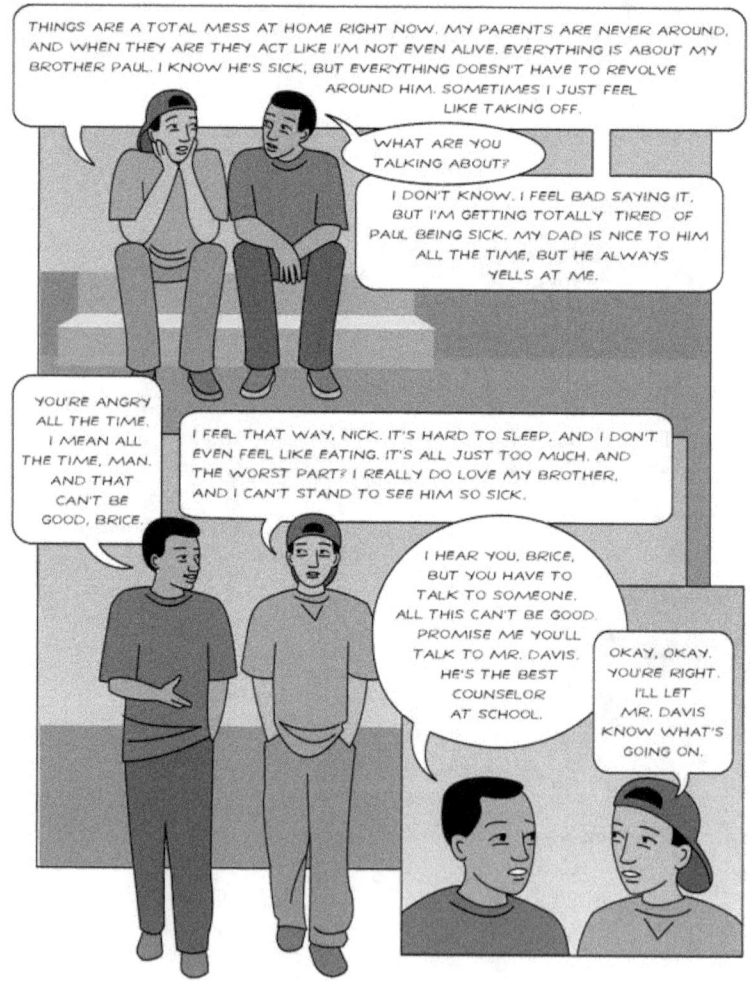

THINGS ARE A TOTAL MESS AT HOME RIGHT NOW. MY PARENTS ARE NEVER AROUND, AND WHEN THEY ARE THEY ACT LIKE I'M NOT EVEN ALIVE. EVERYTHING IS ABOUT MY BROTHER PAUL. I KNOW HE'S SICK, BUT EVERYTHING DOESN'T HAVE TO REVOLVE AROUND HIM. SOMETIMES I JUST FEEL LIKE TAKING OFF.

WHAT ARE YOU TALKING ABOUT?

I DON'T KNOW. I FEEL BAD SAYING IT, BUT I'M GETTING TOTALLY TIRED OF PAUL BEING SICK. MY DAD IS NICE TO HIM ALL THE TIME, BUT HE ALWAYS YELLS AT ME.

YOU'RE ANGRY ALL THE TIME, I MEAN ALL THE TIME, MAN. AND THAT CAN'T BE GOOD, BRICE.

I FEEL THAT WAY, NICK. IT'S HARD TO SLEEP, AND I DON'T EVEN FEEL LIKE EATING. IT'S ALL JUST TOO MUCH. AND THE WORST PART? I REALLY DO LOVE MY BROTHER, AND I CAN'T STAND TO SEE HIM SO SICK.

I HEAR YOU, BRICE, BUT YOU HAVE TO TALK TO SOMEONE. ALL THIS CAN'T BE GOOD. PROMISE ME YOU'LL TALK TO MR. DAVIS. HE'S THE BEST COUNSELOR AT SCHOOL.

OKAY, OKAY. YOU'RE RIGHT. I'LL LET MR. DAVIS KNOW WHAT'S GOING ON.

Why Go to a Counselor?

Remember—going to a counselor means you have the courage to recognize that you're going through a tough time and need some help. Simply put: talking to a counselor can help you feel better. Counselors are specially trained to help you sort out your feelings, gain new skills to deal with what's going on, and find solutions that work for you. Teens who've talked with a counselor say it helped to talk to someone outside their circle of friends and family who didn't take sides, who they could trust. Others say they learned a lot about themselves and felt better able to face life's challenges.

"It took a few visits, but then I got to know and trust my counselor. She really listened to me and was like a coach who helped me learn new skills and see new ways of looking at things. I grew a lot."
—Samantha, age 15

"I was having a really hard time dealing with my sister's cancer. But I tried to be 'perfect' and pretend that everything was okay. I didn't want to stress my parents out even more. One day my aunt said it might help to talk with a counselor—even if it seemed like I had it all together. I was nervous at first, but I went. The counselor made me feel like I could tell her anything—and I finally opened up about how I was really feeling. It felt great to just have someone focus on me and what I was going through." —Jen, age 16

Finding a Counselor

There are many ways to find a counselor. Here are some suggestions to get you started:

→ Talk to your parents or someone else that you trust. Let them know you would like help to get through this difficult time. Tell them that you would like to talk to a counselor. Ask for help making appointments and getting to visits. Sometimes you can even bring a friend.

→ Ask a nurse or social worker at the hospital if they can give you the name of someone you can talk to.

→ Ask your guidance counselor or school nurse if you can talk to him or her.

Joining a Support Group

A good outlet for connecting with teens that are going through the same thing that you are is a support group. Some groups meet in person; others meet online. Some groups go out and do activities together. At first this may not sound like 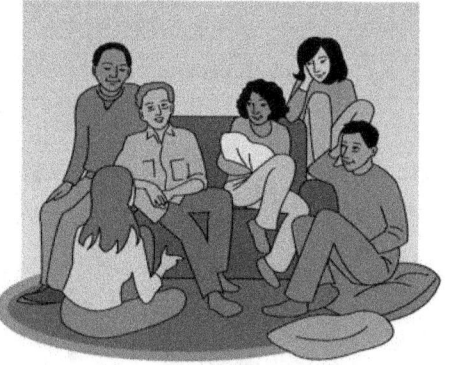 something you want to do. Other teens have thought the same thing—until they went to a meeting. They were surprised that so many other kids felt the same way they did and had advice that really seems to work. Your parents or another trusted adult can help you find a support group.

The best thing about the future is that it comes

Chapter 11

After Treatment

When your brother or sister has finally completed treatment, you and your family may feel a whole range of emotions. Part of you is glad it is over. Another part of you may miss the freedom or new responsibilities you had while your parent was busy taking care of your sick brother or sister.

"My sister Dana had to go to a cancer treatment center 6 hours away. I only got to see her two times. We talked on the phone, but it wasn't the same. My sisters and I sent photos and letters so she knew we were thinking about her. We're glad to have Mom and Dana back home now." —Kyle, age 13

Your brother or sister may still look sick and be weaker than you expected. You may be afraid the cancer will come back. You may be looking to find more meaning in your life now. All these feelings are normal. Things may not go back to exactly how they were before cancer came into your lives. Getting back to your "old life" may take a long time—and it may not happen as you expect.

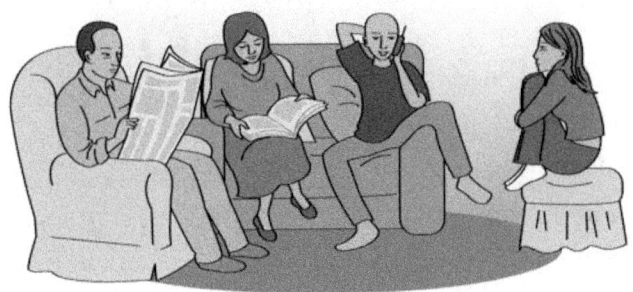

only one day at a time. –Abraham Lincoln

Here's what others have said about life after treatment. Do any of these kids sound like you?

Neil talks about the "new normal":

"I watched my younger brothers when Alex was away getting treatment. My stepdad counted on me since he was working and Mom was at the hospital with Alex all the time. Now that Alex is home, I'm back to being just one of the kids. Alex is getting all the attention—even from my little brothers who used to look up to me all the time. My stepdad says I'll get used to being a kid again. But right now it doesn't feel that way." —Neil, age 16

Ross appreciates life more:

"It used to be all about having the latest stuff. If one of my friends got a new skateboard or jacket, I had to have it, too. After Jackie got sick, I realized that it was just that—stuff. Now there are more important things in life— like my sister and my family. When someone you care about is really sick, you find out what really matters." —Ross, age 15

Tanya is glad to have her sister back home:

"*Before my sister Amy got sick, we fought all the time. If she wore one of my sweaters, I was on her. It bugged me when she followed me around, especially when my friends were over. And if she got into my stuff—it was war. But after Amy got cancer things just didn't matter anymore. I was like—'take my sweater Ames—keep it, it's yours.' I realized how much I would miss her if anything happened to her.*" —Tanya, age 15

Write down what life after treatment feels like for you and your family:

_____

_____

_____

_____

_____

_____

_____

_____

_____

What If Treatment Doesn't Help?

If treatment doesn't help your brother or sister, you and your family will face even more challenges. Hearing that your sibling might die is very difficult. You may feel many of the same emotions you felt when you first learned that your brother or sister had cancer.

No booklet can give you all the answers or tell you exactly how you will feel. But when the future is so uncertain, teens say that it helps to:

→ **Make the most of the time you have.**
Do special things as a family. At home, make time for your brother or sister. Call and visit as much as you can if they are in the hospital. Write notes and draw pictures. Say "I love you" often. If possible, try to have some special times together. If you have not gotten along in the past, you may want to let your brother or sister know you love them.

→ **Stay on track.**
When people get bad news, they often feel like they're living outside of themselves—that life is moving along without them. That's why it's important to keep a schedule and stay connected. Stay involved in school. Be with friends. And let yourself take breaks from it all when you need to.

→ **Have hope.**
Never stop believing in tomorrow, and don't be too hard on yourself. There is more good than bad in this world—even though you might not feel that way right now.

When it is dark enough,

→ **Get help when you feel alone.**
Make sure you find people who can help you. In addition to your family, it may help to talk to a social worker, counselor, or people in a support group. It's important to let your feelings out.

Do you want more support and guidance?

Many cancer organizations can help you during this very difficult time in your life. Turn to Chapter 13 for information about some of these organizations.

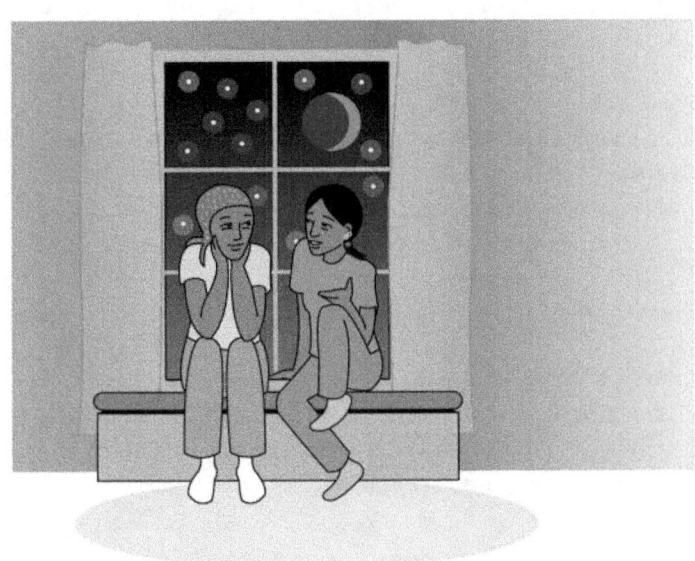

you can see the stars. —Ralph Waldo Emerson

If Your Brother or Sister Passes Away, Know That:

You'll always have memories.
Your brother or sister will always be part of your life. Hold on to your memories of the good times. It's okay to think about something funny that your brother or sister did or said. By laughing and smiling you are bringing back just a little of what was so special about them.

The pain will lessen with time.
At first the pain may be so strong that you might wonder whether you will ever feel happy again. Time has a way of healing. Not being sad every day doesn't mean that you have forgotten. It just means that you're starting to heal.

Everyone grieves in his or her own way.
Some teens grieve for their brother's or sister's death by crying. Others get quiet and spend time by themselves. Some find that they need to be around friends and talk. Others get very angry. In any case, most people finds it helps to keep a regular routine. There is no right or wrong way to grieve. It's okay to deal with loss at your own pace.

Your sibling would want you to be happy.
Stay open to new experiences. Make small changes that give your life new meaning. Write about your thoughts and about this experience. Don't worry about what to say, just write.

Life will change.
Life won't be the same as before, but it can be rich and full again. Keep believing this.

"We all huddled in my mom's bed the night we found out that Gracie's treatment wasn't working anymore. Gracie was so wise. Even though she was only 10 years old, she was trying to comfort us and tell us it would all be okay. That made us want to cry harder—but something inside said to be brave for Gracie. Now, we look at photos and talk about Gracie. I still don't know how life without my little sister will look. I just try to take it one day at a time." —Gail, age 19

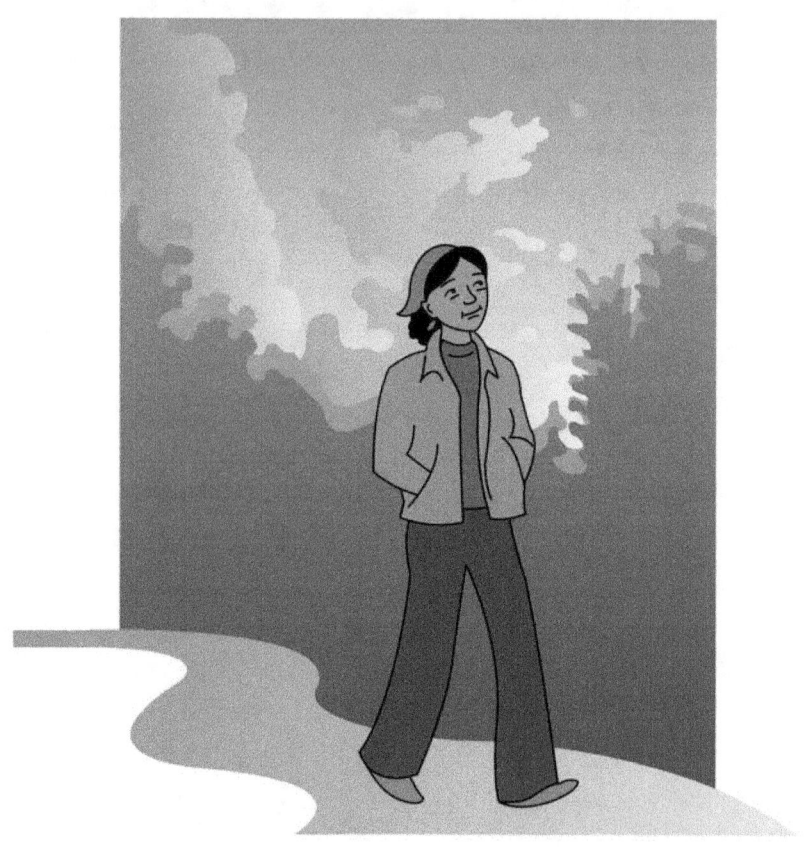

The journey of a thousand miles

    must begin with a

        single step.

           —Lao Tzu

Chapter 12

The Road Ahead

Sometimes things do work out as you hope.

Christine shares her story:

"My brother has been in remission for two years now. Things were pretty bad at first. Then after a while, things sort of settled down and got back to the way they were before. I think Rob's cancer brought us all closer together. I get along better with him and my sister and even with my older brother now. I'm closer to Mom and Dad. And I think we all grew up a lot while he was sick." —Christine, age 15

Sometimes things look like they won't work out as you hope.

Here's what Sam has to say:

"Watching my little brother play with his cars one morning made me so sad. He loves those things. He looked up and told me if he dies I can have all his cars. Then he just went on playing. I felt a huge lump in my throat. He's an amazing little kid." —Sam, age 14

It can be hard to stay calm when you aren't sure what the future holds. You may be thinking—will my brother or sister live? Will the cancer come back? Will life ever be the same? Will I laugh again? Enjoy being with friends again?

While no one can know the future, there are things you can do to make your life a little easier:

→ **Keep talking and pulling together as a family.** You may find that cancer has drawn you closer together and made you appreciate each other more.

→ **Discover your own needs.** Don't let others tell you how you should feel. Allow yourself to cope at your own pace and in your own way.

→ **Remember that you're growing as a person.** Many teens say that having a brother or sister with cancer has made them more sympathetic, more responsible, and stronger.

→ **Keep in mind that you aren't alone.** Right now you may feel lonelier than you ever have in your life. But you are not alone. Family members, friends, neighbors, support groups, and counselors are there to lend a helping hand, listen to you, and give you good advice. Accept their help; you deserve it.

→ **Appreciate each day.** Many teens who have a brother or sister with cancer say that they learned to see the world more clearly. In time you may come to appreciate things you may have overlooked in the past.

Maybe you have noticed that little things seem to have more meaning for you these days. Take some time to write these thoughts down, even if they seem small:

_____

_____

_____

_____

_____

_____

_____

_____

_____

_____

_____

_____

Unfortunately, no booklet or person can tell you how everything is going to work out. Cancer is tough, and your life may never be quite the same. But in the end, you will get through it. Why? You're strong. And you are capable—even if you don't always feel that way.

It's great that you want to learn more!

Keep in mind that cancer treatments are getting better all the time. Make sure that what you read or see is up to date and accurate. Talk with your parents or another trusted adult about what you find. Share the articles or books you've found with them. Ask them any questions you may have.

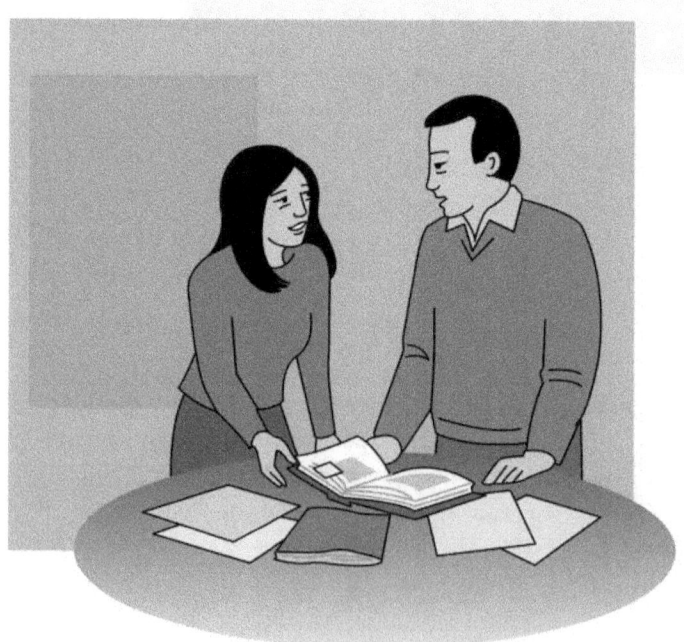

Chapter 13

Learning More on Your Own

Your school or public library

Ask the librarian to help you find the information or support that you're looking for in books, magazines, videos, or on the Internet.

The Internet

Use an Internet search engine and type in general words like "sibling" and "cancer" together to get started. Keep in mind that the Internet has a lot of good information. It also has a lot of poor information and false promises, so you may want to check with your parent or another trusted adult about what you find.

Your sibling's hospital or clinic

Visit the patient education office at your sibling's hospital, if there is one. Or, ask if you can go with your brother or sister during their visit to the doctor to learn more.

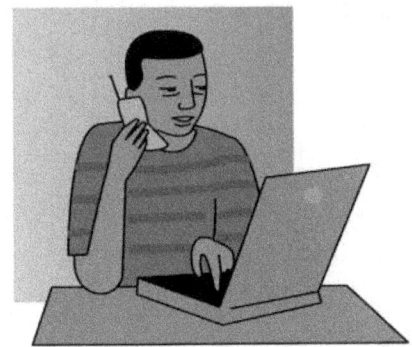

Help Is a Phone Call or Web Site Away

Here are some places to contact for help. You can call them or visit their Web site for more information.

National Cancer Institute (NCI)
Cancer Information Service (CIS)
1-800-4-CANCER (1-800-422-6237)
www.cancer.gov

NCI offers accurate, up-to-date information on cancer for you and your family. Call the CIS to talk to an information specialist who can answer questions you or someone in your family might have. Or go to LiveHelp on NCI's Website to chat online with an information specialist. NCI can also help connect you with a support organization in your area. NCI offers many materials in both English and Spanish. People who are deaf may call a special TTY line at 1-800-332-8615.

American Camp Association
1-800-428-2267
www.acacamps.org

The American Camp Association can help you find camps that are specifically for kids who have a brother or sister with cancer.

American Cancer Society (ACS)
1-800-ACS-2345 (1-800-227-2345)
www.cancer.org

By calling ACS, you can talk to a cancer information specialist. You can call 24 hours a day to get your questions answered. The specialist may help you find information and other resources.

CancerCare
1-800-813-HOPE (1-800-813-4673)
www.cancercare.org

CancerCare offers free information and support by telephone and online to anyone affected by cancer. Visit their online support group for teens who have a brother or sister with cancer.

Candlelighters Childhood Cancer Foundation
1-800-366-CCCF (1-800-366-2223)

www.candlelighters.org

Candlelighters Childhood Cancer Foundation provides support, education and advocacy for children and adolescents with cancer, survivors of childhood/adolescent cancer, their families and the professionals who care for them.

Gilda's Club
1-800-GILDA-4-U (1-800-445-3248)

www.gildasclub.org

Gilda's Club provides a place for people with cancer and their families and friends to join with others to build social and emotional support. They offer support groups, workshops, and social activities for people affected by cancer. Call to see whether there is a location near you.

Make-A-Wish Foundation
1-800-722-WISH (1-800-722-9474)

www.wish.org

Make-A-Wish grants wishes to kids who have life-threatening medical conditions. Your parents, your brother or sister with cancer, or their doctor can call Make-A-Wish to see whether your brother or sister can qualify.

SuperSibs!
1-866-444-SIBS (1-866-444-7427)

www.supersibs.org

SuperSibs! is a national non-profit organization that provides free services to brothers and sisters of children with cancer. SuperSibs! helps children and teens redefine the "cancer sibling" experience by providing them with ongoing recognition and support.

The Wellness Community
1-888-793-WELL (1-888-793-9355)

www.thewellnesscommunity.org

The Wellness Community offers support, education, and hope to people with cancer and their loved ones. Call to find out whether there is a location near you.

91

Appendix

Chart A: Monitoring Tests

TEST	PURPOSE
Biopsy	Used to find out whether a tumor or abnormality is cancer. Benign means it is not cancer. Malignant means that it is cancer.
Blood test	Checks the blood to see whether the balance of the cells and chemicals is normal
Bone marrow aspiration	Collects a small sample of cells from inside a bone to be examined under a microscope
CAT scan or CT scan (Computerized axial tomography)	Uses x-rays and a computer to produce three-dimensional (3-D) images of the inside of the body
MRI (Magnetic resonance imaging)	Uses radio and magnetic waves to make images of organs and other tissues inside the body
PET scan (Positron emission tomography)	Uses computerized pictures of areas inside the body to find cancer cells
Spinal tap (Lumbar puncture)	Collects a sample of the fluid inside the spine to be examined under a microscope
Ultrasound (Ultrasonography)	Uses high-frequency sound waves to make images of internal organs and other tissues inside the body
X-ray	Takes a picture of the inside of the body using high-energy waves

PROCEDURE (What Happens)

A doctor removes a sample from a person using one of two ways: with a long needle (needle biopsy) or by making a small cut (surgical biopsy).

A nurse or technician inserts a needle into a vein, usually in the arm. Then he or she draws blood.

A needle is used to remove a small sample of tissue from a bone (usually the hip bone).

The patient lies flat on a table, which moves through a large tube while a series of x-rays is taken.

The patient lies flat on a table, which moves through a large tube while an MRI machine scans the body for several minutes.

The patient gets an injection and then a machine takes computerized pictures of areas inside the body.

A needle is used to remove fluid from the spine in the lower back.

A technician moves a small handheld device over an area on the patient's body. An image appears on the computer screen.

The patient is placed in front of the x-ray machine or lies on a table.

Chart B: Cancer Team Members

TEAM MEMBER	WHAT THEY DO
Child life specialist	A trained person who works with children and their families to make the hospital and treatment experience less scary
Nurse	A health professional trained to care for people who are ill or disabled
Nutritionist/ dietitian	A health professional with special training in nutrition who can help with dietary choices
Oncologist	A doctor who specializes in treating people with cancer. Some oncologists specialize in certain types of cancer or certain types of cancer treatment
Patient educator	Educates patients and families about illness
Pharmacist	Dispenses medicines for patients
Physical therapist	Teaches exercises and physical activities that help patients gain more muscle strength and movement
Psychiatrist	A doctor who treats mental health problems, including depression, with medicine and talk therapy
Psychologist	Talks with patients and their families about emotional and personal matters and helps them make decisions, but does not write prescriptions for medicines
Radiologist	A doctor who looks at x-rays and other images of the body
Religious or spiritual leader	Addresses the spiritual and emotional health of patients and their families. This can be a chaplain, minister, priest, rabbi, imam, or youth group leader
Social worker	Talks with people and their families about emotional or physical needs and helps them find support services
Surgeon	A doctor who removes or repairs a part of the body by operating on the patient

Glossary

What the Terms Mean

This list can help you learn some words that your parents or the doctors and nurses may use. Don't be afraid to ask questions when you don't understand what they are talking about. These people are there to help you, too.

Benign: Not cancer. Benign tumors do not spread to the tissues around them or to other parts of the body.

Biological therapy: Treatment to help the body's immune system fight infections, cancer, and other diseases. It is also used to reduce certain side effects of cancer treatment. Other names include immunotherapy, biotherapy, or BRM (biological response modifier) therapy.

Bone marrow: The soft, sponge-like tissue in the center of most bones. It makes white blood cells, red blood cells, and platelets.

Cancer: A term for diseases in which abnormal cells divide without control. Cancer cells can invade nearby tissues and can spread through the bloodstream and lymphatic system to other parts of the body.

These are the main types of cancer:

- **Carcinoma** starts in the skin or in tissues that line or cover internal organs.

- **Leukemia** starts in blood-forming tissue such as the bone marrow. Large numbers of abnormal blood cells form and enter the bloodstream.

- **Lymphoma** and **multiple myeloma** begin in the cells of the immune system.

- **Sarcoma** starts in bone, cartilage, fat, muscle, blood vessels, or other connective or supportive tissue.

Cell: The individual unit that makes up all the tissues of the body. All living things are made up of cells.

Chemotherapy or **chemo:** Treatment with medicines that kill cancer cells. Chemo is most often given intravenously (through a blood vessel). Some chemo can also be given by mouth.

Clinical trial: A type of research study that tests how well new medical approaches work in people. These studies test new methods of screening, prevention, diagnosis, or treatment of a disease.

Depression: A mental condition marked by ongoing feelings of sadness, despair, loss of energy, and difficulty dealing with normal daily life. Other symptoms of depression include feelings of worthlessness and hopelessness, loss of pleasure in activities, changes in eating or sleeping habits, and thoughts of death or suicide. Depression can affect anyone, and can be successfully treated.

Diagnosis: Identifying a disease by its signs and symptoms.

Donor: A person whose stem cells match with those of the person with cancer. Not everyone is a match. A patient's brother or sister is more likely to match than someone who is not related.

Hormone: A chemical made by glands in your body. Hormones move in the bloodstream. They control the actions of certain cells or organs.

Hormone therapy: Treatment that uses hormones to slow or stop the growth of certain cancers such as prostate and breast cancer.

Immune system: Organs and cells that defend the body against infections and other diseases.

Intravenous or **IV:** Injected into a blood vessel.

Leukemia: Cancer that starts in blood-forming tissue such as the bone marrow and causes large numbers of blood cells to form and enter the bloodstream.

Malignant: Cancerous. Cells from a malignant tumor can enter and destroy nearby tissue and spread to other parts of the body.

Metastasis: The spread of cancer from one part of the body to another. A tumor formed by cells that have spread is called a metastatic tumor or a metastasis.

Protocol: A plan for treating cancer.

Radiation therapy: Treatment with high-energy radiation to kill cancer cells and shrink tumors. External radiation comes from a machine outside the body. Internal radiation comes from material put inside the patient near the cancer cells.

Recurrence: The return of cancer after a period when it seemed to be gone. The cancer may come back in the same place as the first time or in another place in the body. Also called recurrent cancer.

Relapse: The return of signs or symptoms of cancer after a period of improvement.

Remission: During remission, the signs and symptoms of cancer go away or are less than before. In partial remission, some, but not all, signs and symptoms of cancer have disappeared. In complete remission, all signs and symptoms of cancer have disappeared, although cancer may still be in the body.

Sibling: Another way of saying your brother or sister.

Side effects: Problems that can occur when cancer treatment harms healthy tissues or organs. Some common side effects of cancer treatment are feeling tired, pain, being sick to the stomach, vomiting, lower blood cell counts, hair loss, and mouth sores.

Stem cells: Cells from which other types of cells develop. For example, blood cells develop from blood-forming stem cells.

Stem cell transplantation: The use of healthy stem cells from the bone marrow or the bloodstream to replace cells that were destroyed by high doses of chemotherapy and/or radiation therapy. The transplanted stem cells may come from the patient or from donors. In many cases, the donors are family members. The patient gets the stem cells through an IV line.

Support group: A group of people with similar concerns who help each other by sharing experiences, knowledge, and information.

Surgery: An operation to remove or repair a part of the body.

Tissue: A group or layer of cells that work together to perform a specific function.

Transfusion: The infusion of certain blood cells or whole blood into the bloodstream. The blood may be donated from another person, or it may have been taken from the patient earlier and stored until needed.

Transplant: The replacement of tissue with tissue from the patient's own body or from another person.

Tumor: A mass of tissue that forms when cells divide more than they should or do not die when they should. A tumor may be cancerous (malignant) or not cancerous (benign).

X-ray: A type of high-energy radiation. In low doses, x-rays are used to spot diseases by making pictures of the inside of the body. In high doses, x-rays are used to treat cancer.

Make a list of any terms that still aren't clear to you. Talk to your parents, doctors, nurses, or other adult about your questions.

Acknowledgments

We would like to thank the many teens, scientists, and health professionals who assisted with the development and review of this publication.

To know the road ahead,

ask those coming back.

--Chinese proverb